BC Cancer Agency

~~Cancer Centre~~

D0379192

WITHDRAWN

Randomised Controlled Trials

Randomised Controlled Trials

A user's guide

Alejandro R Jadad,

Director, McMaster Evidence Based Practice Center Co-Director, Canadian Cochrane Network and Centre Health Information Research Unit Department of Clinical Epidemiology and Biostatics Faculty of Health Sciences, McMaster University, Hamilton, Canada

© BMJ Books 1998
BMJ Books is an imprint of the BMJ Publishing Group

All rights reserved. No part of this publication may be reproduced,
stored in a retrieval system, or transmitted, in any form or by any
means, electronic, mechanical, photocopying, recording and/or
otherwise, without the prior written permission of the publishers.

First published in 1998
by BMJ Books, BMA House, Tavistock Square,
London WC1H 9JR

British Library Cataloguing in Publication Data

A catalogue record for this book is available from the
British Library

ISBN 0-7279-1208-9

Typeset, printed and bound in Great Britain by
Latimer Trend & Company Ltd, Plymouth

Contents

Foreword

Around 600 BC, Daniel of Judah conducted what is probably the earliest recorded clinical trial. He compared the health effects of a vegetarian diet with those of a royal Babylonian diet over a ten day period.[1] Despite the dramatic findings of the study, over four centuries elapsed before publication of the results. The trial had obvious deficiencies by contemporary methodologic standards (allocation bias, ascertainment bias, confounding by Divine intervention),[2] but the publication has remained influential for over two millennia.

Other controlled clinical studies with methodologic weaknesses but important effects on practice have been undertaken during the ensuing centuries. Ambrose Paré (1514–1564), in an unplanned experiment, found that applying a soothing "digestive medicament" to battle wounds produced better results than the traditional practice of cauterising wounds with boiling oil.[3] Inoculation to prevent smallpox became popular after Maitland conducted a trial upon six Newgate convicts in 1721,[3] although the numbers treated and the precision of the trial were not adequate to give a fair picture of the effects of the procedure. Jenner published his famous studies on vaccination at the end of the eighteenth century, based on 10 and 14 persons. Appalled by the ravages of scurvy among ships crews on long voyages, in 1747 James Lind conducted a comparative trial of the most promising scurvy cures, using as subjects 12 sick seamen on board the *Salisbury* at sea. "The most sudden and visible good effects were perceived from the use of the oranges and lemons." The British Navy did not supply lemon juice to its ships until 1795.[3]

The nineteenth century saw many major advances. Probably the most sophisticated trial of a preventive type was a before/after study conducted by Ignaz Semmelweis in 1847. He noted that maternal mortality was much higher among women delivered by physicians and medical students, who were in frequent contact with cadavers at autopsies, than among women delivered by pupil midwives. After considering various hypotheses he reasoned that "the cadaveric particles clinging to the hands are not entirely removed by the ordinary method of washing the hands", and introduced the practice of more thorough washing and disinfectant.[4] Maternal mortality among the doctor-delivered mothers dropped by 50 per cent in the subsequent six months, although still not to as low a level as that achieved by the midwives.

Credit for the modern randomised trial is usually given to Sir Austin Bradford Hill. The historic MRC trials on streptomycin for pulmonary tuberculosis[5] are rightly regarded as a landmark that ushered in a new era of medicine. Their influence on the science of therapeutic evaluation was strengthened because the charismatic Hill followed up that work with lectures and articles[6] reinforcing his message. Since Hill's pioneer achievement randomised trial methodology has been increasingly accepted, and the number of randomised controlled trials reported has grown exponentially. The Cochrane Library[7] already lists more than 150,000 such trials, and they have become the underlying basis for what is currently called "evidence based medicine". The concept has rightly been hailed as a paradigm shift in our approach to clinical decision making.[8]

It is not, however, the first such paradigm shift. A similar scientific revolution was hailed more than a century and a half ago, by the editor of the *American Journal of Medical Sciences* in 1836, in his introduction to an article which he considered to be "one of the most important medical works of the present century, marking the start of a new era in science". It was "the first formal exposition of the results of the *only true method of investigation* (emphasis added) in regard to the therapeutic value of remedial agents". The article that evoked such effusive praise was the French study on blood-letting in the treatment of pneumonia by PCA Louis.[9,10]

At that time blood-letting was the almost universally accepted "proper" method of treating pneumonia. Louis used the quintessential Baconian approach of gathering vast amounts of data, which allowed him to make comparisons and systematically investigate the efficacy of treatments. His conclusion from that study was a bombshell; that the apparent efficacy of bleeding for pneumonia was a mere therapeutic illusion. His contribution to clinical epidemiology was to base recommendations for therapy on the results of collective experience, rather than on limited individual experience, tradition, or theory.

Louis' approach, and his evangelical zeal in promoting his methods created considerable controversy. He attracted many foreign disciples, including Oliver Wendell Holmes and William Osler who made their mentor's work available to American readers. He also attracted strong opposition, and his work was mired in controversy. His opponents were numerous and vociferous: "The physician called to treat a sick man is not an actuary advising a company to accept or deny risks, but someone who must deal with a specific individual at a vulnerable moment" and "Averages could not help and might even confuse the practising physician as he struggles to apply general rules to a specific case." Practising physicians were unwilling to hold their decisions in abeyance till their therapies received numerical approbation, nor were they prepared to discard therapies validated by both tradition and their own experience on account of somebody else's numbers.[10]

Although doubtless they arose partly from an innate resistance to change, and partly from misguided self-interest, the arguments against a widespread application of the so-called numerical approach stemmed largely from a lack of understanding of its intent. When both practitioners and public finally became aware that collective experience enhanced, rather than replaced, the clinical skills of the individual physician, Louis' numerical approach became the basis of medical research and literature until the midpoint of this century. It was by no means a panacea, but was an enormous step on the way towards more effective health care.

The arguments heard against the numerical approach in the last century are remarkably similar to those used against evidence based medicine today. Worries are still being expressed that evidence based medicine confuses statistics with reality, results in a loss of clinical freedom, and ignores the importance of clinical experience and of individual values.[11] These concerns stem from the mistaken belief that the proponents of evidence based medicine claim a multicentre double blind placebo controlled randomised trial to be the only way to answer a therapeutic question. This, despite the fact that Austin Bradford Hill himself said "Any belief that the controlled trial is the only way would mean not that the pendulum had swung too far, but that it had come right off its hook".[12] Evidence based medicine is simply the conscientious and judicious use of the current best evidence from clinical care research to guide health care decisions. It is another enormous step towards more effective health care. No more, and no less.

One reason for the sometimes expressed opposition to evidence based medicine is a lack of understanding of the meaning of a randomised trial. This failure of understanding is not due to a paucity of information; there is a vast literature about randomised trials, their purpose, their methodology, their limitations. Unfortunately, much of that literature has been incomplete, has been biased, or has been couched in impenetrable jargon. It is not surprising that it has often been misinterpreted.

That is why this book is so welcome. It is written in clear, explicit, and understandable language, for those who use, would like to use, or should use, the results of randomised trials. It provides an accurate and comprehensive description of the randomised trial, its importance, when (and when not to) do a trial, how to interpret the results, when (and when not to) translate the results into health care decisions. It is a book to read, reflect on, learn from, use, and enjoy.

Murray W. Enkin, MD, FRCS(C)

Professor Emeritus, Departments of Obstetrics and Gynaecology, and Clinical Epidemiology and Biostatistics, McMaster University, Canada.

1 Book of Daniel. In: The Holy Bible.
2 Grimes D. Clinical research in ancient Babylon: methodologic insights from the book of Daniel. *Obstet Gynecol* 1995;**86**:1031–4.
3 Bull BP. The historical development of clinical therapeutic trials. *J Chron Dis* 1959;**10**:218–243.
4 Semmelweis I. *The etiology, the concept, and the prophylaxis of childbed fever* (1861).Translated by Carter KC. University of Wisconsin Press. 1983.
5 Daniels M, Hill AB. Chemotherapy of pulmonary tuberculosis in young adults: an analysis of the combined results of three medical research council trials. *Br Med J* 1952; **1**:1162–8.
6 Hill AB. The clinical trial. *New Eng J Med* 1952;**247**:113–19.
7 *The Cochrane Library*. Oxford: Update Software. 1998, issue 1.
8 Evidence-based Medicine Working Group. Evidence-based medicine: a new approach to teaching the practice of medicine. *JAMA* 1992;**268**:2420–25.
9 Louis PCA. 'Researches into the effects of blood-letting in some inflammatory diseases and on the influence of tartarized antimony and vesication in pneumonitis. *Am J Med Sci* 1836;**18**:102–11 (cited in Rangachari 1997).
10 Rangachari PK. Evidence-based medicine: old French wine with a new Canadian label? *J Royal Soc Med* 1997;**90**:280–4.
11 Charlton BG. Restoring the balance: evidence-based medicine put in its place. *J Eval Clin Pract* 1997;**3**:87–98.
12 Hill AB. Heberden oration, 1965. Reflections on the controlled trial. *Ann Rheum Dis* 1966;**25**:107–13.

Introduction

This is a book for busy readers who need, wish or have to understand the basic principles of randomised controlled trials (RCTs) and their role in health care decisions. It is my best effort to fill a gap in the literature that I was not able to fill with any single source during the past 15 years.

In the 1980s, as a medical student, intern, resident, and novice researcher, I could not find a single source that could help me really understand what RCTs were about, their strengths and limitations, and how to use them while making health care decisions. During that decade, I had to rely on many sources, most of which had been written in a language that was difficult for me to understand, that presented information in formats that I could not adapt to my busy life or to my rapidly changing needs. I attributed my failed attempts to find a single, easy-to-read source of basic information to the fact that I was in Colombia, a developing country where it was often difficult to access the biomedical literature.

In 1990 I moved to Oxford, England, where I spent 5 years as a research fellow, as a practising clinician and as a graduate student. At the beginning of this period, the need for a good source of information to fill my most basic knowledge gaps intensified. My colleagues at Oxford were seasoned trialists. They not only designed and analysed their own trials, but also criticised, quite strongly, RCTs done by others. As I did not want to bother my colleagues with basic questions (or to sound dumb), I started looking, again, for a source of information that could meet my most immediate needs. To my surprise, I could not find one. I started to list my questions and decided to get answers as soon as possible, from as many sources as necessary. I spent vast amounts of time (and not insignificant amounts of money) trying to get small pieces of information from different books, most of which targeted doers of research, not users. I also started asking for key references from colleagues, and tracked down articles mentioned by speakers at conferences or included in the reference lists of the articles I was collecting from other sources. As my list of questions grew, so did my list of references and contacts. After a while, I felt more comfortable to talk to my colleagues about trials, started to design and lead some trials myself, and was invited to coordinate journal club sessions, where the work of others was rigorously appraised. Two years after my arrival in Oxford, one of my RCTs was published in the *Lancet!* This experience, however, created a new set of challenges. Colleagues started to invite me to give lectures on pain research and trial design. I found myself under a different type of pressure. I had the opportunity, for the first time, to transmit to others what I had learnt. I began to feel confident about acknowledging my own uncertainties and knowledge gaps. People seemed to like my presentations and I started to receive invitations to give lectures. It did not take me long to realise that the attendees were asking similar questions from lecture to lecture, and that those questions were similar to those I had listed before. I started recording the questions and made every effort to address them during each successive lecture. Soon, some of the new questions from the audience started to coincide with my own questions at the time. I kept adding any new questions to my list for the five years I was in England. The questions I collected, approximately 100, form the backbone of this book.

In 1992, I was accepted as a graduate student at the University of Oxford and started to work on a thesis on meta-analysis of randomised trials in pain relief. As part of my thesis work, I coded over 15 000 citations and created a database with over 8 000 RCTs. I also led the development of what is regarded by many as the first validated tool to appraise the quality of RCTs, and created new statistical methods to combine data from different RCTs addressing the same topic. When I tried to use the newly developed methods to answer clinical important questions, I realized that despite having thousands of RCTs at my fingertips, relevant data were often unavailable or poorly reported. I also started to formulate questions around RCTs that had not yet been answered at all and became interested in the design of methodological studies to answer them. During this period, I started to meet people who shared my interest in addressing unanswered methodological questions. Most of them had published a number of studies that looked at the RCT as the subject of research, rather than as the research tool. Through my interaction with this different breed of researchers and their work, and my own methodological studies, I became aware of how vulnerable the RCT can be to bias, imprecision, irrelevance and politics at all stages of its development and in all areas in health care.

Soon after I completed my thesis work, I moved to McMaster University, where I expected to have a quieter time, as a postdoctoral fellow, applying all my new knowledge on RCTs and systematic reviews, and exploring ways to involve consumers in health decisions. I was pleasantly surprised. I found lots of exciting work on RCTs and systematic reviews at McMaster; but through my interaction with my new colleagues, I became aware of the profound influence that factors other than evidence from RCTs can have on clinical decisions and health outcomes. Under their influence, I began to grasp the complexity of human–human, human–information, human–technology and information–technology interactions. My world became richer, and once again I faced new challenges. I started to look on RCTs as powerful but vulnerable tools that can make important but small contributions to a large puzzle with many pieces that are continuously changing their shape, size and patterns.

At that point, writing a book on RCTs moved from being a relatively easy task to a daunting one. I almost turned down the offer to write this book. It took me more than a year to draft the first chapter, and more than another year to complete the book.

At first, I was tempted to target the book to both doers (i.e. fellow researchers and academics) and users (i.e., clinicians, policy makers and managers, and if brave enough, consumers) of research. After drafting many tables of contents, I realized that trying to meet the needs of such a diverse group at the same time would be a mistake. After some deliberation, I decided to produce an introductory guide for busy readers. Primarily, this book is aimed at clinicians, young researchers, research staff and trainees in any health profession. Nevertheless, I hope that health planners, managers, journal editors, peer-reviewers, journalists, members of consumer advocacy groups and even seasoned researchers could also find it relevant and useful.

The book is divided into eight chapters, and addresses 100 questions with short answers and key references. The first five chapters focus on individual trials and include definitions of key elements of trials, descriptions of different types of RCTs and sources of bias, discussions of different approaches to quality assessment, and tips on trial reporting and interpretation. The sixth chapter focuses on groups of RCTs and includes discussions on different types of reviews, meta-analyses and clinical practice guidelines. The seventh chapter addresses the role of RCTs in health care decisions, their relationship with the other types of information, values, preferences and circumstances. This chapter also introduces the basic principles of evidence based decision-making and highlights its strengths and limitations. The last chapter describes "my wish list". In it, I highlight what I think are the most important barriers to the optimal use of RCTs in health care, and propose some strategies that could be used to overcome them.

Writing each of the chapters of this book was an extraordinary experience, full of challenges and lessons. The main challenge was to ensure that I could complete the book without affecting my family life or my responsibilities as a new faculty member. The only way in which I could do this was by modifying my sleep pattern. This book was written, essentially, from 11 pm to 2 am or from 4 am to 6 am. Working at these hours gave me more time than I had had in years to think about trials and to put together my thoughts without interruptions. Putting each chapter together forced me to be concise and to use easy-to-read language to describe even the most complex aspects of RCTs. I made every effort to describe the key elements and implications of RCTs without statistics, and in a way that would appeal to busy readers. Each chapter created new questions and opened new avenues for me to explore. During each session I struggled, continuously, to keep the balance between the need to describe the basic elements of RCTs and the urge to express my concerns and expectations about health care research as a whole.

In sum, I did my best to provide you with an enjoyable, basic, balanced, useful and broad view of RCTs and their role in health care. I hope I succeeded.

Alejandro (Alex) R. Jadad
Dundas, 11 June 1998

Acknowledgments

I would like to express my gratitude to all those, now anonymous, who asked me most of the questions that provided the structure of this book.

I would also like to thank a group of special people who have contributed significantly to my education as a clinician, researcher and teacher over the past ten years. During my training in Colombia, Mario Ruiz exerted great influence on my research life, introduced me to the joy of clinical research and taught me the indelible meaning of the word mentor. German Parra showed me, for the first time, how research evidence can be integrated into clinical decisions, and Pedro Bejarano encouraged me, selflessly, to develop my research career abroad.

In England, Henry McQuay showed me the power of RCTs in health care and provided me with unprecedented conditions to nurture my curiosity and to speed up the development of my research skills. Iain Chalmers introduced me to systematic reviews and exemplified the meaning of collaboration. Chris Glynn showed me that busy clinicians can be researchers, provide humane patient care and have a rich personal life beyond medicine. His continuous challenges encouraged me to see the limitations of research evidence to guide health care decisions and motivated many of my efforts to overcome them. Clive Hahn encouraged me to write this book and Mary Banks, Senior Commissioning Editor at BMJ Books made sure that it happened.

This book would have been much different without the influence of many of my colleagues at McMaster University. Some of them deserve special mention. I owe a lot to George Browman, who created the opportunity for me to come to Canada, expanded my research horizons, helped me to recognise the value of the research process and other types of information, and gave me unconditional support to develop my own agenda. I would also like to thank Brian Haynes, for reinforcing my notion of mentorship, and for helping me understand the need to integrate research evidence with the values, preferences and circumstances of the decision-makers. Geoff Norman introduced me to the principles of cognitive and social psychology, opened my eyes to the limitations of human inference, encouraged me to focus the book on users of research, and challenged me continuously to recognise the barriers to the practice of evidence based decision-making created by our human nature.

For advice on matters academic or personal, I have turned repeatedly to Murray and Eleanor Enkin, my favourite couple. My family and I feel immensely privileged to call them friends. We owe them a great deal for the warmth with which they have welcomed us into their lives, for their wisdom, and for the kind but always-candid advice. Murray read each of the chapters of this book, and gave me invaluable advice on both content and structure. Each contact with Murray and Eleanor, regardless of whether it centres around academic, family or cultural issues, is always a rich learning experience.

I would also like to express my gratitude to those who gave their time to me generously to help put this book together. Tracy Hillier, Geoff Norman and Iain Chalmers provided very constructive comments on the initial outline of the book.

Susan Marks read, patiently, each of the chapters of the book, always giving me friendly and highly professional suggestions to improve their readability and structure. Judi Padunsky proofread most of the chapters, supported my communication with the publishers and organised the references for the entire book. Laurie Kendry and Mary Gauld read several chapters of the book and provided valuable input. Comments by Brian Haynes and Geoff Norman contributed enormously to the last chapter.

I owe more to my family than to anyone else. My extended family in South America showed me, from a very early age, the meaning of teamwork, unconditional support and trust. I could not have possibly written this book without Martha, my wife and best friend. Once more, her love, support and constructive criticism have helped me maintain a busy academic life and be part of a happy family. Finally, I would like to give special thanks to my daughters Alia and Tamen, for giving a new meaning to all I do.

To my family

Questions

Chapter 4: Assessing the quality of RCTs: why, what, how and by whom?

Chapter 5: Reporting and interpreting individual trials: the essentials

Chapter 8: My wish list: thinking it all over

1 Randomised controlled trials: the basics

What is a randomised controlled trial?

The randomised controlled trial (RCT) is one of the simplest, most powerful and revolutionary tools of research.[1,2] In essence, the RCT is a study in which people are allocated at random to receive one of several clinical interventions.

The people who take part in RCTs are called participants or study population (or, less politically correct, "subjects"). Participants do not necessarily have to be ill, because as the study can be conducted in healthy volunteers, in relatives of patients, or in members of the general public. The people who design the study, administer the interventions, assess the results, and analyse them are called the investigators. The interventions are also called clinical manoeuvres, and include actions of such varied natures as preventive strategies, diagnostic tests, screening programmes and treatments. For instance, in a study in which patients with rheumatoid arthritis are randomised to receive either ibuprofen or a new non-steroidal anti-inflammatory drug (let's call it "perfectafen") for the relief of pain, you and your colleagues are the investigators, the participants are the patients with rheumatoid arthritis, and the interventions are ibuprofen and the new drug, perfectafen.

Typically, RCTs seek to measure and compare different events that are present or absent after the participants receive the interventions. These events are called outcomes. As the outcomes are quantified (or measured), RCTs are regarded as quantitative studies. In the RCT comparing ibuprofen and perfectafen, for instance, the investigators could select pain as the main outcome, measuring it in terms of the number of patients who achieve complete relief one week after starting treatment. Also, because RCTs are used to compare two or more interventions, they are considered to be comparative studies. You should be aware that there are other types of studies that may be quantitative but do not include comparisons among groups (that is, case series). These studies are also known as non-comparative studies (see Chapter 7).

Usually, one of the interventions is regarded as a standard of comparison or control, and the group of participants who receive it is called the control group. This is why RCTs are referred to as randomised *controlled* trials. The control can be conventional practice, a placebo, or no intervention at all. The other groups are called the experimental or the treatment groups. In the example, the experimental group is the group that receives perfectafen and the control group is the one that receives ibuprofen.

RCTs are experiments because the investigators can influence the number and the type of interventions, as well as the regimen (amount, route, and frequency) with which the interventions are applied to the participants. I mention this because there is another group of studies in which the events are measured but not influenced by the investigators (they are called observational), and others in which the researchers do not even measure events, but try to interpret them in their natural settings (these studies are called qualitative). Other types of studies are described in more detail in Chapter 7.

In summary, RCTs are quantitative, comparative, controlled experiments in which a group of investigators studies two or more interventions in a series of individuals who receive them in random order.

Are the elements of RCTs very different from other studies?

Apart from random allocation to the comparison groups, the elements of an RCT are no different from the components of any other type of prospective, comparative, quantitative study. These components include the rationale and objectives of the study, the research question that the investigators hope to answer, the methodology used to answer it, the results of the study, and its conclusions. These components will be discussed in the following four chapters.

What does random allocation mean?

Random allocation means that all participants have the same chance of being assigned to each of the study groups.[3] Therefore, allocation is not determined by the investigators, the clinicians, or the study participants.

Despite its simplicity, the principle of randomisation is often misunderstood by clinicians, researchers, journal reviewers and journal editors. It is therefore important for you to be aware that methods for allocating participants according to date of birth (odd or even years), the number of their hospital records, the date at which they are invited to participate in the study (odd or even days), or alternatively into the different study groups, do not give each of the participants the same chance to be included in each of the study groups. Therefore, they should not be regarded as methods that generate random allocation sequences. These methods are often described as "pseudo-random" or "quasi-random". The main problem associated with these methods is that knowledge of the group to which a participant is assigned can affect the decision about whether to enter him or her into the trial and this can bias the results of the whole trial.[3,4] If no one cheats, however, these studies could produce well balanced groups. As discussed in Chapter 3, sequences generated randomly can also be subverted easily.

The studies that use pseudo-random or quasi-random methods of allocation are also known as a non-randomised controlled trials. Together with RCTs, these trials form a group of studies called controlled clinical trials. In fact, the RCT is also known as a randomised *clinical* trial. In other words, all RCTs are controlled clinical trials, but not all controlled clinical trials are RCTs.

What is the purpose of random allocation?

By allocating the participants randomly, the characteristics of the participants are likely to be similar across groups at the start of the comparison (also called the baseline). If this is the case, the groups are called balanced at baseline. By keeping the groups as similar as possible at the start of the study, the investigators will be more able to isolate and quantify the impact of the interventions that they are studying, with minimal effects from other factors that could influence the course of the study participants. The factors that could influence the outcomes of a study, which are not related directly to the interventions, could be known or unknown. For instance, randomisation can balance the proportion of patients taking antacids in the study comparing ibuprofen with perfectafen.

3

Although keeping the groups balanced in terms of known factors is important, it can also be achieved without randomisation, as long as the factors have been measured. For example, if perfectafen is evaluated in a retrospective study, the investigators can select a group of patients who received ibuprofen and took antacids which would match the proportion of patients who took antacids and received perfectafen.

In summary, the real value of randomisation is that, if it is done properly, it reduces the risk of serious imbalance in unknown but important factors that could influence the clinical course of the participants. No other study design allows investigators to balance these unknown factors.

You must understand that the risk of imbalance among the groups is not abolished completely, even if the allocation is perfectly randomised. There are many types of bias that can influence the composition and characteristics of the study groups. These biases are discussed in Chapter 3.

How can randomisation be achieved?

The generation of random sequences of allocation can be achieved using one of a variety of procedures. Regardless of the method used, investigators should follow two rules: first, they must define the rules that will govern allocation; and, second, they should follow those rules strictly throughout the whole study.

The simplest methods to generate random sequences of allocation are flipping a coin (for studies with two groups) or rolling a die (for studies with two or more groups). As mentioned, the first step is to define the allocation rules. For instance, before flipping a coin, investigators may decide that the tails would correspond to group A and the heads to group B. In addition, when rolling a die in a study with two groups, investigators can choose to allocate participants to group A with odd numbers and to group B with even numbers. With three groups, they can choose to allocate participants to group A if the die shows 1 or 2, to group B if 3 or 4, and to group C if 5 or 6. And so on. Instead of dice or coins, investigators can also use other simple methods such as drawing balls of different colours or ballots with the study group labels from a dark bag.

Investigators can also use random number tables or computers to generate the sequences. Random number tables are tables that contain a series of numbers which occur equally often and are arranged in a random (therefore unpredictable) fashion. The numbers usually have two or more digits. The use of a random number table forces investigators to make more choices than with a coin or a die. As with the coin or the die, they must first decide the correspondence between the numbers and the groups (that is, odd corresponding to A and even to B; or numbers from 00 to 33 to group A, from 34 to 66 to group B, and from 67 to 99 to group C). Then, they have to select the starting point in the table (that is, the beginning, the end, or any point in the middle of the table marked by a pencil dropped with the eyes closed) and the direction in which the table will be read (that is, upwards or downwards). If the numbers in the table contain more than two digits, the investigators have to select the position of the numbers that will determine allocation. For example, if the table contains numbers with four digits (that is, 2314), the investigators can choose the last two digits (14), the first two (23), the second (3), the last (4), the first (2) or the last three (314). The crucial issue is that, once the procedure is defined, it is not modified at any point during the study.

A similar set of numbers may be generated by a computer that is programmed to do so or by most scientific calculators. The procedures and rules that the investigators must follow are identical to those described for the random number tables.

Regardless of the method chosen by the investigators to generate random sequences of allocation, the number and characteristics of the participants allocated to each of the study groups will probably differ (although slightly) at any given point during the study.[3] To minimise these differences, investigators can use some strategies known as restricted (or block) randomisation or stratified randomisation.

Restricted randomisation is used to keep the numbers of participants in all the study groups as close as possible. It is achieved by creating "blocks" of sequences which will ensure that the same number of participants will be allocated to the study groups within each block. For example, in a study with three groups (A, B, and C), the investigators can create six blocks: ABC, ACB, BAC, BCA, CAB, CBA. If they use a die to generate the sequences, then they can decide how each of the six numbers of the die will correspond to each of the blocks. In this case, however, each of the sequences will determine the allocation of three participants at the same time, not only one at a time. For instance, if it is decided that 1 corresponds to the sequence ABC, then the three participants that enter the study after a die has shown 1 will be allocated in that order: the first participant to group A, the second to group B, and the third to group C. Equally, if 2 corresponds to ACB, then the first participant to be included in the study after the die shows 2 will be allocated to group A, the second to group C, and the third to group B. The blocks can be of any size, but ideally the size should correspond to a multiple of the number of groups in the study (that is, six blocks for a study with two or three groups).[3]

Stratified randomisation is used to keep the characteristics of the participants (that is, age, weight, or functional status) as similar as possible across the study groups. To achieve this, investigators must first identify factors (or strata) that are known to be related to the outcome of the study. Once these factors are identified, the next step is to produce a separate block randomisation scheme for each factor to ensure that the groups are balanced within each strata.

On occasion, investigators may not desire the same number of participants in each of the study groups and can decide to allocate unequal numbers to each group, while preserving the homogeneity of the distribution of the characteristics of the participants across the study groups. This is called weighted or unequal randomisation. This type of randomisation tends to be used by investigators who wish to expose fewer participants to the experimental group because of concerns about unexpected adverse events. In the example of ibuprofen versus perfectafen, the investigators may decide to allocate one patient to perfectafen for each four patients who receive ibuprofen.

Unfortunately, the methods of allocation in studies described as "randomised" are poorly and infrequently reported, even when such studies are published in prominent journals.[5,6] As a result of these poor descriptions, it is not possible to determine, on most occasions, whether the investigators used a proper method to generate random sequences of allocation.

On the other hand, when the reports of studies described as randomised provide details of the methods of allocation, it has been shown that 5–10% do not use methods that generate random sequences.[7,8]

The reporting of randomisation and other aspects of RCTs will be discussed in detail in Chapter 5.

What can be randomised in RCTs?

The most frequent unit of allocation in RCTs is individual people, either patients (the most common) or caregivers (that is, treating physicians or nurses).

Sometimes, however, it is more appropriate to randomise groups of people rather than individuals. This is known as cluster randomisation. Examples of these groups or clusters are hospitals, families, and geographical areas. Investigators frequently use this approach when the RCTs are designed to evaluate interventions that may affect more than one individual within a particular group (that is, an RCT evaluating the effect of a videotape on smoking cessation on prison inmates or the effects on parents following early discharge from hospital after childbirth). It is also used when the way in which the participants in one study group are treated or assessed is likely to modify the treatment or assessment of participants in other groups. This phenomenon is known as contamination. For example, contamination is present in an RCT comparing a booklet with strategies to increase patient participation in treatment decisions versus conventional practice, if clinicians who have given the booklet to a group of participants start using the strategies described in the booklet during the treatment of participants who do not receive the booklet.

In other cases, investigators may decide to randomise not only individuals or groups of individuals, but also the order in which the measurements are obtained from each participant. For instance, in an RCT evaluating the effects of morphine on cancer pain, the investigators could randomise the order in which analgesia, adverse effects, and quality of life are assessed.

Can RCTs answer all clinical questions?

Although RCTs are considered "the best of all research designs"[9] or "the most powerful tool in modern clinical research",[10] they are not a panacea to answer all clinical questions. There are many situations in which they are not feasible, necessary, appropriate, or even sufficient to help solve important problems.

RCTs are the ideal study design to answer questions related to the effects of health care interventions which are small to moderate. The term "intervention" is widely used in health care, but infrequently defined. On most occasions the term "intervention" refers to treatment. As discussed at the beginning of this chapter, however, this term should be used in a much wider sense to include any clinical manoeuvre offered to the study participants that may have an effect on their health status (that is, preventive strategies, screening programmes, diagnostic tests, the setting in which health care is provided, or educational models).

Even though RCTs are appropriate to evaluate health care interventions, you must be aware that there are many important issues in health care that could be studied by RCTs, but for which there are no RCTs available. In addition, even when RCTs are available, they may be insufficient to provide all the answers required by clinicians, patients, or policy makers.[11,12] In these cases, you will have to wait for more RCTs to be completed, do more RCTs yourself, or use other types of studies either as your only source of research information or as a complement to the information provided by RCTs. Other study designs and other types of information, with their advantages and disadvantages, are discussed in Chapter 7.

There are also questions for which RCTs are not appropriate. These are usually questions related to aspects of health care that cannot or should not be influenced by the investigators. These include issues related to the aetiology or natural history of diseases. It would be inappropriate, for instance, to design an RCT in which people would be randomised to smoke or not to smoke for decades to compare the frequency of lung cancer between smokers and non-smokers.

In other circumstances, RCTs may not be appropriate even to study some interventions. For example, it may be unfeasible (particularly because of financial constraints, low compliance rates, or high drop out rates) to design an RCT to evaluate the effects of interventions with very rare outcomes or with effects that take long periods of time to develop. In these cases, other study designs such as case–control studies or cohort studies are more appropriate.

The corollary is that, before you start reading an RCT, or even searching for one, you should take into account that there are other study designs that may be more appropriate than an RCT to answer your particular questions (a brief description of studies other than RCTs is provided in Chapter 7). Even if an RCT is available, you must be aware that one RCT in isolation, even when it is appropriate and perfectly designed, is unlikely to provide all the answers that you need. You should consider the information provided by a single RCT as an important piece in a puzzle with many empty spaces. This information will have to be assessed and used in conjunction with other types of information (for example, data from other RCTs or from other study designs, and your own clinical experience), and the values and preferences of the people involved in the decisions, depending on the circumstances in which the decisions are being made.

1 Silverman WA, Chalmers I. Sir Austin Bradford Hill: an appreciation. *Controlled Clin Trials* 1992;**13**:100–5.
2 Jadad AR, Rennie D. The randomized controlled trial gets a middle-aged checkup. *JAMA* 1998;**279**: 319–20.
3 Altman DG. *Practical statistics for medical research*. London: Chapman & Hall, 1991.
4 Schulz KF, Chalmers I, Hayes RJ, Altman DG. Empirical evidence of bias: dimensions of methodological quality associated with estimates of treatment effect in controlled clinical trials. *JAMA* 1995;**273**:408–12.
5 Altman DG, Doré CJ. Randomisation and baseline comparisons in clinical trials. *Lancet* 1990;**335**:149–53.
6 Moher D, Fortin P, Jadad AR, Jüni P, Klassen T, Le Lorier J, Liberati A, Linde K, Penna A. Completeness of reporting of trials in languages other than English: implications for the conduct and reporting of systematic reviews. *Lancet* 1996; **347**:363–6.
7 Mosteller F, Gilbert JP, McPeek B. Reporting standards and research strategies for controlled trials: agenda for the editor. *Controlled Clin Trials* 1980;**1**:37–58.
8 Evans M, Pollock AV. Trials on trial: a review of trials of antibiotic prophylaxis. *Arch Surg* 1984;**119**:109–13.
9 Norman GR, Streiner DL. *Biostatistics: the bare essentials*. St Louis: CV Mosby, 1993.
10 Silverman WA. Gnosis and random allotment. *Controlled Clin Trials* 1981;**2**: 161–4.
11 Naylor CD. Grey zones of clinical practice: some limits to evidence-based medicine. *Lancet* 1995;**345**:840–2.
12 Freemantle N. Dealing with uncertainty: will science solve the problem of resource allocation in the UK NHS? *Soc Sci Med* 1995;**40**:1365–70.

2 Types of randomised controlled trials

Randomised clinical trials (RCTs) can be used to evaluate different types of interventions in different populations of participants, in different settings, and for different purposes. Once investigators ensure that allocation of participants to the study groups is random (to call the study an RCT), they can design the study using strategies to match the characteristics of the interventions they want to study, the resources they have available, and their academic, political, marketing, or clinical motivations.

Over the years, multiple terms have been used to describe different types of RCTs. This terminology has evolved to the point of becoming real jargon. This jargon is not easy to understand for those who are starting their careers as clinicians or researchers, because there is no single source with clear and simple definitions for all these terms.

In this chapter, I will describe the most frequent terms used to describe different types of RCTs. I will do my best to classify them in a way that will be easy for you to follow, understand, and remember. Some of the terms apply specifically to RCTs, whereas others may also be applied to other study designs. Some terms are mutually exclusive, some overlap considerably, and some complement each other. On occasion, I will include terms that are used to describe other types of studies that are not necessarily RCTs, to ensure that you are aware of the differences between them.

RCTs can be classified according to: (1) the aspect of the interventions investigators want to explore; (2) the way in which the participants are exposed to the interventions; (3) the number of participants included in the study; (4) whether the investigators and participants know which intervention is being assessed; and

---

Box 2.1 Different types of RCTs

RCTs according to the aspects of the interventions they evaluate

- Explanatory and pragmatic trials
- Efficacy and effectiveness trials
- Phase I, II, and III trials

RCTs according to how the participants are exposed to the interventions

- Parallel trials
- Crossover trials
- Trials with factorial design

RCTs according to the number of participants

- From n-of-1 to mega-trials
- Fixed size
- Sequential trials

RCTs according to whether the investigators and participants know which intervention is being assessed

- Open trials
- Single blind trials
- Double blind trials
- Triple and quadruple-blind trials

RCTs according to whether the preferences of non-randomised individuals and participants are taken into account

- Zelen's design
- Comprehensive cohort design
- Wennberg's design

---

(5) whether the preferences of non-randomised individuals and participants are taken into account in the design of the study (Box 2.1).

RCTs that explore different aspects of the interventions

Depending on the aspects of the interventions that investigators want to evaluate, RCTs can be classified as: explanatory or pragmatic; as efficacy, effectiveness, or equivalence trials; and as phase I, II or III.

What is the difference between explanatory and pragmatic trials?

Explanatory trials address whether or not an intervention works. If the intervention works, then these trials attempt to establish how such intervention works. Typically, these trials are designed in such a way that the results are likely to yield a "clean" evaluation of the interventions. To achieve this, the investigators set strict inclusion criteria that will produce highly homogeneous study groups. For instance, investigators designing an explanatory study of the effects of a new antihypertensive drug could decide to include only patients aged between 40 and 50 years, with no coexisting diseases (that is, diabetes) and exclude those receiving other particular interventions (β-blockers).

Explanatory trials also tend to use placebos as controls, fixed regimens (that is, 20 mg by mouth every 6 hours), long washout periods (if patients have been taking diuretics, for instance, those drugs will be stopped for a sufficient period of time to ensure that they are "washed out" of their bodies), intention to treat analysis (see Chapter 3), and focus on "hard" outcomes (that is, blood pressure recorded at specific times after a detailed and standardised process).

Pragmatic trials (also called management trials) are designed not only to determine whether the intervention works, but also to describe all the consequences of its use, good and bad, under circumstances mimicking clinical practice.[1] To achieve this, pragmatic studies tend to use more lax criteria to include participants with heterogeneous characteristics, similar to those seen by clinicians in their daily practice. In addition to the more lax inclusion criteria, pragmatic trials tend to use active controls (that is, the new antihypertensive drug vs a β-blocker), flexible regimens (that is, 20 mg orally every 6 hours, reducing or increasing the dose by 5 mg according to the degree of blood pressure control and adverse effects), and analysis of the patients who received the interventions (see Chapter 3). Pragmatic trials do not preclude the use of "soft" outcome measures, such as measures of sexual function or quality of life.

Although both explanatory and pragmatic approaches are reasonable and even complementary, it is important that you understand that they represent the extremes of a spectrum and that most RCTs include a combination of elements from each. The key issue is whether the investigators achieved the best combination of elements to answer their (and your) questions.

What is the difference between efficacy and effectiveness?

RCTs are often described in terms of whether they evaluate the efficacy or the effectiveness of an intervention. These two concepts are frequently misunderstood.

Efficacy refers to whether an intervention works in people who receive it.[2] Trials designed to establish efficacy (also called efficacy trials) tend to be explanatory trials, because they are designed to yield a "clean" evaluation of the effects of the intervention. In this particular case, however, the investigators are not so interested in finding out how the intervention works. Instead, their main goal is to include participants who will follow their instructions and who will receive the intervention. The extent to which study participants follow the instructions given by the investigators is called compliance or adherence. High compliance is easy to achieve when the administration of the interventions is completely controlled by the investigators or by other health professionals, who are not acting as investigators but are supportive of the study (that is, an RCT evaluating the effects of coronary artery bypass surgery and those of angioplasty in patients with unstable angina). This is more difficult when the interventions are not administered by the investigators but by the participants themselves, when the study has a long duration, and when the interventions have to be administered several times a day. Returning to the example of the antihypertensive drug discussed in the previous section, compliance will depend on the extent to which the participants take the antihypertensive tablets as prescribed for the whole duration of the study. The investigators in charge of this study may choose to include patients who have already shown high compliance in other studies.

Effectiveness refers to whether an intervention works in people to whom it has been offered.[2] These RCTs, also called effectiveness trials, tend to be pragmatic, because they try to evaluate the effects of the intervention in circumstances similar to those found by

13

clinicians in their daily practice. The design of effectiveness trials is usually simpler than the design of efficacy trials, because effectiveness trials tend to follow lax inclusion criteria, include flexible regimens, and allow participants to accept or reject the interventions offered to them. Typically, effectiveness trials evaluate interventions with proven efficacy when they are offered to a heterogeneous group of people under ordinary clinical circumstances.

On occasions, trials are designed not to detect possible differences in efficacy or effectiveness between two or more interventions, but to show that the interventions are, within certain narrow limits, "equally effective"[3] or equally efficacious. These trials are called equivalence trials. Often, these trials seek to demonstrate that a new intervention (or a more conservative one) is at least as good as the conventional standard treatment. Investigators who engage in equivalence trials make efforts to minimise the risk of suggesting that the interventions have equivalent effects when in fact they do not. Strategies to minimise this type of risk are described in Chapters 3 and 4.

What are phase I, II and III trials?

These terms are used to describe the different types of trials that are conducted during the evaluation of a new drug. Phase I and II trials are not usually randomised.

As the name suggests, phase I trials are the first studies conducted in humans to evaluate a new drug. Phase I trials are conducted once the safety and potential efficacy of the new drug have been documented in animals. As the investigators know nothing about the effects of the new drug in humans, phase I trials tend to focus primarily on safety. They are used to establish how much of a new drug can be given to humans without causing serious adverse effects, and to study how the drug is metabolised by the human body.[4] Phase I trials are mostly conducted on healthy volunteers. The typical participant in a phase I study is one of the investigators who developed the new drug, either an employee of a pharmaceutical company or a member of a research team at a university. People with diseases for which there is no known cure (that is, AIDS and certain types of cancer) often participate in phase I trials. As mentioned above, these trials are often not randomised, and not even controlled. Usually, they are just series of cases in which the participants are given incremental doses of the drug, without a control group, while they are monitored carefully by the investigators. In addition to the inherent limitations of case series, the main problem of this type of trial is that, if the participants are patients, those who are studied at the beginning are likely to receive very low doses which are unlikely to be effective, whereas those studied later are at greater risk of receiving toxic doses but are also more likely to benefit if the drug is effective.

After the safety of a new drug has been documented in phase I trials, investigators can proceed to conduct phase II trials. These are trials in which the new drug is given to small groups of patients with a given condition (usually about 20 per trial). The aim of phase II trials is to establish the efficacy of different doses and frequencies of administration. Even though phase II trials focus on efficacy, they can also provide additional information on the safety of the new drug. Often, phase II trials are not randomised, particularly when the therapeutic effects of the new drug can be measured objectively. For instance, if a new drug has been designed to treat a type of cancer that is associated with a high mortality rate, the investigators will conduct a phase II trial in which about 20 patients will receive the drug while tumour response, mortality and adverse effects are monitored carefully. If the drug is judged to be ineffective or excessively toxic, no more trials will be conducted. If the drug produces a good response (that is, "fewer patients than expected" die), however, and patients tolerate its adverse effects, the investigators can proceed to a phase III trial. When the effects of the new drug are assessed using subjective measures (that is, pain relief with a new analgesic drug), the investigators can use a randomised design in which they will compare the effects of the new drug with a placebo (see below) to ensure that the effects observed in the small groups of patients can be attributed to the new drug and not to other factors (that is, a placebo effect).

Phase III trials are designed and conducted once a new drug has been shown to be reasonably effective and safe in phase II trials.[4] Phase III trials are typically effectiveness trials, because they seek to compare the new drug with an existing drug or intervention known to be effective. This existing drug is usually regarded as the current standard treatment.[4] Most phase III trials are RCTs.

There is an additional group of studies called phase IV trials. The term "phase IV trial" is used to represent large studies[3] that seek to monitor adverse effects of a new drug after it has been

15

approved for marketing.[4] These studies are also called postmarketing surveillance studies. They are mostly surveys and seldom include comparisons among interventions.[3] The term "phase IV trial" can also be used to describe promotional strategies to bring a new drug to the attention of a large number of clinicians.[4] In either case, phase IV trials are not RCTs.

RCTs according to the participants' exposure to the interventions

Depending on the extent to which the participants are exposed to the study interventions, RCTs can have parallel, crossover, or factorial designs.

What is a parallel design?

Most RCTs have a parallel design. In these studies (also called parallel trials or RCTs with parallel group design), each group of participants is exposed to only one of the study interventions. For instance, if a group of investigators uses a parallel design to evaluate the effects of a new analgesic compared with those of a placebo in patients with migraine, they would give the new analgesic to one group of patients and placebo to a different group of patients.

What is a cross-over design?

An RCT has a cross-over design when each of the participants is given all the study interventions in successive periods. The order in which the participants receive each of the study interventions is determined at random. Crossover trials produce *within* participant comparisons, whereas parallel designs produce *between* participant comparisons. As each participant acts as his or her own control in crossover trials, they can produce statistically and clinically valid results with fewer participants than would be required with a parallel design.[5]

The time during which each of the interventions is administered and evaluated is called a period. The simplest crossover design includes only two periods. Returning to the example of the new analgesic, if the same group of investigators uses a crossover design, they would randomise each patient to receive the new analgesic first and then the placebo, or vice versa—the placebo first and then the new analgesic.

Crossover trials are not always appropriate. Every time you read the report of a crossover trial, you should explore the extent to which some basic rules are followed.

The interventions should be used in chronic, incurable diseases

Patients who are cured by one or more of the interventions will not be eligible to enter subsequent periods of a crossover trial. This means that the ability of the crossover trial to produce within patient comparisons is lost and the baseline characteristics of the participants in each period are no longer the same. Ignoring this rule can bias the results of a crossover trial substantially, particularly when a crossover trial is used to compare the effects of a drug that can cure a disease with those of a placebo[6] (see Chapter 3).

The effects of interventions should have rapid onset and short duration

This minimises the risk of drop out within each period and helps to keep the number of participants stable across periods. In addition, if the effects of the intervention are of short duration, they are less likely to persist during the administration and evaluation of another intervention.

When the effects of an intervention are still present during the evaluation of another, such effects are called carry-over effects. If any observed difference between the interventions can be explained by the order in which the interventions were given to the participants, this is called a treatment-period interaction and it can invalidate the trial. Carry over effects can be predicted when the duration of the effects of the interventions are well known. In these cases, carry over effects can be prevented by separating the study periods by a period of time of sufficient length to enable the participants to be free of the influence of the intervention previously used by the time they receive the next intervention.[3] This amount of time is also known as a washout period.

The condition (or disease) must be stable

If the disease is stable, the circumstances at the beginning of each period are more likely to be the same than if the disease is not stable. For instance, a crossover design to evaluate the new analgesic will produce more valid results in patients with migraine than in patients with postoperative pain because the intensity of postoperative pain tends to decrease with time. Even if the new analgesic was studied only in patients with migraine, the results of a crossover trial would be more valid if it included patients who have suffered similar episodes of migraine for many years than in patients who present episodes of migraine of different and unpredictable duration or intensity. All the differences between the study periods that are caused by disease progression, regression, or fluctuation are called period effects.

Carry over and period effects are known as order effects. Both can be assessed and removed from the comparisons by using statistical manoeuvres that are beyond the scope of this book, but that are described elsewhere.[7]

What is a factorial design?

An RCT has a factorial design when two or more experimental interventions are not only evaluated separately, but also in combination and against a control. For instance, a factorial design to study the effect of an opioid (that is, morphine) and a non-steroidal anti-inflammatory drug (that is, ibuprofen) for the treatment of cancer pain would mean that patients will be allocated randomly to receive ibuprofen only, morphine only, a combination of morphine and ibuprofen, or placebo. This design allows the investigators to compare the experimental interventions with the control (that is, morphine vs placebo), compare the experimental interventions with each other (that is, morphine vs ibuprofen), and investigate possible interactions between them (that is, comparison of the sum of the effects of morphine and ibuprofen given separately with the effects of the combination).

RCTs according to the number of participants

RCTs can include from one to tens of thousands of participants, they can have fixed or variable (sequential) numbers of participants, and they can involve one or many centres.

Is it possible for an RCT to have only one participant?

The answer is yes. These RCTs are called "n-of-1 trials" or "individual patient trials". Basically, they are crossover trials in which one participant receives the experimental and the control interventions, in pairs, on multiple occasions and in random order. These trials provide individual, rather than generalisable, results. They can be very useful when it is not clear whether a treatment will help a particular patient. You may find yourself in this situation, for instance, when you have a patient with a rare disease and there are no trials supporting the use of the treatment in that particular disease, or when the patient does not have a rare disease, but the treatment has been evaluated in studies that include very different patients.[8] Typically, the number of pairs of interventions varies from two to seven. Usually, the number of pairs is not specified in advance, so that the clinician and the patient can decide to stop when they are convinced that there are (or that there are not) important differences between the interventions.

The success of n-of-1 trials to guide clinical decisions depends largely on whether the patient is willing to collaborate and on whether the rules described in relation to crossover trials (see above) are followed. A detailed description of how to design, conduct, and analyse n-of-1 trials is beyond the scope of this book, but can be found elsewhere.[9]

What is a mega-trial?

"Mega-trial" is a term that is being used increasingly to describe RCTs with a simple design (usually very pragmatic) which include thousands of patients and limited data collection.[10,11] Usually, these trials require the participation of many investigators (sometimes hundreds of them) from multiple centres and from different countries. The main purpose of these large simple trials is to obtain "increased statistical power" and to achieve wider generalisability. This means that their aim is to increase the chances of finding a difference between two or more interventions, if such a difference exists. This issue will be discussed in more detail in Chapter 5.

What is a sequential trial?

A sequential trial is a study with parallel design in which the number of participants is not specified by the investigators beforehand. Instead, the investigators continue recruiting participants until a clear benefit of one of the interventions is observed, or until they are convinced that there are no important differences between the interventions.[12] These trials allow a more efficient use of resources than trials with fixed numbers of participants, but they depend on the principal outcome being measured relatively soon after trial entry.

What is a fixed size trial?

In a fixed size trial the investigators establish deductively the number of participants (also called sample size) that they will include. This number can be decided arbitrarily or can be calculated using statistical methods. The main goal of using statistical methods to calculate the sample size is to maximise the chance of detecting a statistically and clinically significant difference between the interventions when a difference really exists (see Chapter 5).

RCTs according to whether the investigators and participants know which intervention is being assessed

In addition to randomisation (which helps control selection bias), the investigators can incorporate other methodological strategies to reduce the risk of other biases. These biases and the strategies to control them will be discussed in detail in Chapter 3. I have brought this issue to your attention in this chapter because the presence, absence, or degree of one of these strategies has been used to classify RCTs. This strategy is known as "blinding" or, perhaps more appropriately (but rarely used), "masking". In clinical trial jargon, blinding or masking represents any attempt made by the investigators to keep one or more of the people involved in the trial (that is, the participant or the investigator) unaware of the intervention that is being given or evaluated. The purpose of blinding is to reduce the risk of ascertainment or observation bias. This bias is present when the assessment of the outcomes of an intervention is influenced systematically by knowledge of which intervention a participant is receiving. Blinding can be implemented at at least six different levels in an RCT. These levels include the participants, the investigators, or clinicians who administer the interventions, the investigators or clinicians who take care of the participants during the trial, the investigators who assess the outcomes of the interventions, the data analysts, and the investigators who write the results of the trial. As you might expect, in many studies those individuals who administer the interventions, take care of the participants, assess the outcomes, or write the reports are the same. Depending on the extent of blinding, RCTs can be classified as open, single-blind, double-blind, triple-blind, and quadruple-blind.

What is an open RCT?

An open RCT is a randomised trial in which everybody involved in the trial knows which intervention is given to each participant. Most trials comparing different surgical interventions or comparing surgery with medication are open RCTs.

What is a single-blind RCT?

A single-blind RCT is a randomised trial in which one group of individuals involved in the trial does not know the identity of the intervention that is given to each participant. Usually it is the participants or the investigators assessing the outcomes who do not know the identity of the interventions. Single blind designs are used frequently to evaluate educational or surgical interventions. For instance, investigators could evaluate different educational strategies in patients who would be unaware of the different types of strategies that are being compared. In addition, two surgical procedures could be compared under single-blind conditions with the use of identical wound dressings to keep investigators blind to the type of procedure during the assessment of the outcomes.

What is a double-blind RCT?

A double-blind RCT is a randomised trial in which two groups of individuals involved in the trial do not know the identity of the intervention that is given to each participant. Usually, these two groups include the participants and the investigators in charge of assessing the outcomes of the interventions.

To be successful, double-blinding requires that the interventions must be indistinguishable to both the participant and the investigator assessing the outcomes. Usually, the interventions are known to them just as A or B. When the experimental intervention is new and there are no standard effective interventions that could be used as controls, the investigators use an inert substance, or placebo, which has the same appearance and taste as the

21

experimental intervention. These double-blind RCTs, in which the control group receives a placebo, are also called double-blind, randomised, placebo controlled trials.

When the RCT is designed to compare a new intervention with a standard treatment, the RCTs are called active-controlled. Achieving double-blinding in active-controlled trials is often difficult and frequently requires the use of what is called a double dummy. In a double-blind, double dummy RCT, each group of participants receives one of the active interventions and a placebo (in this case called a dummy) that looks and tastes the same as the other intervention. The double dummy technique is particularly useful when the investigators want to compare interventions that are administered by different routes or that require different techniques of administration. For instance, a double-blind, double dummy RCT would be the ideal study design to compare one intervention that is given as a tablet with another that is given by injection. In such a trial, the participants in one of the study groups would receive a tablet with the active drug and a placebo injection, whereas the participants in the other group would receive a placebo tablet and an injection with the active drug.

Problems with the way in which double-blinding is implemented, evaluated, and described in RCTs will be discussed in Chapters 3 and 4.

What is a triple-blind or quadruple-blind RCT?

In a triple-blind RCT, three groups of individuals involved in the trial do not know the identity of the intervention that is given to each participant. These groups could include the participants, the investigators giving the intervention, and those evaluating the outcomes (if the latter two are different); or the participants, the investigators evaluating the outcomes, and the data analysts.

If one more group is unaware of the identity of the intervention that is given to each participant, then the trial becomes a quadruple-blind RCT. This could easily be achieved by making the investigators who write the results of the trial unaware of the identity of the interventions until the time at which they complete the manuscript. Even though it is easy to make a double-blind trial into a triple or quadruple-blind trial, it happens very rarely.

RCTs that take into account the preferences of non-randomised individuals and participants

Eligible individuals may refuse to participate in trials, either because they have a strong preference for one particular intervention (if there are several active interventions available) or because they do not want to receive a placebo. Other eligible individuals may decide to participate in a trial despite having a clear preference for one of the study interventions. The outcomes of these individuals, whether they enter the trial or not, may be different from those participants who do not have strong preferences. The outcomes of the individuals who do not participate in the trials or of those who participate and have strong preferences are rarely recorded.

There are at least three types of RCTs that take into account the preferences of eligible individuals, whether they take part in the trial or not. These trials are called preference trials, because they include at least one group in which the participants are allowed to choose their own preferred treatment from among several options offered.[13,14] These trials can have Zelen's design, a comprehensive cohort design, or Wennberg's design (Fig 2.1).

What is a trial with Zelen's design?

In a trial with Zelen's design, eligible individuals are randomised before they give consent to participate in the trial, to receive either a standard treatment or an experimental intervention. Those who are allocated to standard treatment are given the standard treatment and are not told that they are part of a trial, whereas those who are allocated to the experimental intervention are offered the experimental intervention and told that they are part of a trial. If they refuse to participate in the trial, they are given the standard intervention but are analysed as if they had received the experimental intervention.[15]

The main advantages of Zelen's design are that almost all eligible individuals are included in the trial and that the design allows the evaluation of the true effect of offering experimental interventions to patients. The main disadvantages are that they have to be open trials and that the statistical power of the study may be affected if a high proportion of participants choose to have the standard treatment.

23

To overcome the ethical concerns of not telling patients that they have been randomised to receive the standard treatment, the original approach proposed by Zelen can be modified by informing participants of the group to which they have been allocated and by offering them the opportunity to switch to the other group (Fig 2.1a). This design is also known as double randomised consent design.[16] Even though this modified design overcomes the ethical concerns of the original Zelen's design, it does not solve the problems associated with lack of blinding and potential loss of statistical power.[14]

What is a trial with comprehensive cohort design?

A comprehensive cohort trial is a study in which all participants are followed up, regardless of their randomisation status (Fig 2.1b). In these trials, if a person agrees to take part in an RCT, he or she is randomised to one of the study interventions. If the person does not agree to be randomised because he or she has a strong preference for one of the interventions, that person will be given the preferred intervention and followed up as if he or she were part of a cohort study (see Chapter 7).[16,17] At the end, the outcomes of people who participated in the RCT can be compared with those who participated in the cohort studies to assess their similarities and differences.

This type of design is ideal for trials in which a large proportion of eligible individuals are likely to refuse to be randomised because they (or their clinicians) have a strong preference for one of the study interventions.[16] In these cases, it could be said that the study is really a prospective cohort study with a small proportion of participants taking part in an RCT.[16] One of the main limitations of this type of design is that any differences in outcomes may be explained by differences in the baseline characteristics of the participants in the randomised and non-randomised groups.[18,19]

What is a trial with Wennberg's design?

In a trial with Wennberg's design eligible individuals are randomised to a "preference group" or an "RCT group" (Fig 2.1c). Those individuals in the preference group are given the opportunity to receive the intervention that they choose, whereas those in the RCT group are allocated randomly to receive any of

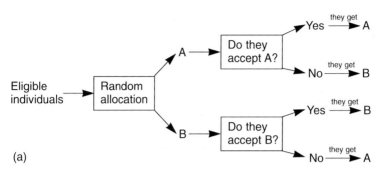

(a)

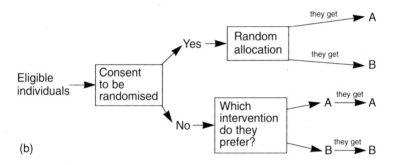

(b)

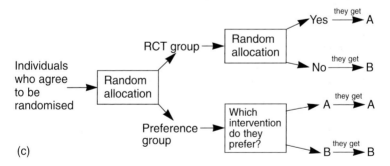

(c)

Figure 2.1 Preference trials: (a) Zelen's design with double randomised consent; (b) comprehensive cohort design; and (c) Wennberg's design.

25

the study interventions, regardless of their preference. At the end of the study, the outcomes associated with each of the interventions in each of the groups are compared and used to estimate the impact of the participants' preferences on the outcomes.

Preference trials are rarely used in health care research. They are, however, likely to become more frequently used as consumer participation in health care decisions and research increases.

1 Sackett DL, Gent M. Controversy in counting and attributing events in clinical trials. *N Engl J Med* 1979;**301**:1410–12.
2 Fletcher RH, Fletcher SW, Wagner EH. *Clinical epidemiology: the essentials*, 3rd edn. Baltimore, MD: Williams & Wilkins, 1996.
3 Armitage P, Berry G. *Statistical methods in medical research*, 3rd edn. Oxford: Blackwell Scientific, 1994.
4 Pocock SJ. *Clinical trials: a practical approach.* Chichester: Wiley, 1983.
5 Louis TA, Lavori PW, Bailar JC III, Polansky M. Crossover and self-controlled designs in clinical research. In: Bailar JC III, Mosteller F, eds. *Medical uses of statistics*, 2nd edn. Boston, MA: New England Medical Journal Publications, 1992:83–104.
6 Khan KS, Daya S, Collins JA, Walter SD. Empirical evidence of bias in infertility research: overestimation of treatment effect in crossover trials using pregnancy as the outcome measure. *Fertil Steril* 1996;**65**:939–45.
7 Senn S. *Cross-over trials in clinical research.* Chichester: John Wiley & Sons, 1993.
8 Guyatt G, Sackett D, Taylor DW, Chong J, Roberts RS, Pugsley S. Determining optimal therapy—randomized trials in individual patients. *N Engl J Med* 1986; **314**:889–92.
9 Sackett DL, Haynes RB, Guyatt GH, Tugwell P. *Clinical epidemiology: a basic science for clinical medicine*, 2nd edn. New York: Little, Brown & Company, 1991.
10 Woods KL. Mega-trials and management of acute myocardial infarction. *Lancet* 1995;**346**:611–14.
11 Charlton BG. Mega-trials: methodological issues and clinical implications. *J R Coll Physicians Lond* 1995;**29**:96–100.
12 Altman DG. *Practical statistics for medical research.* London: Chapman & Hall, 1991.
13 Till JE, Sutherland HJ, Meslin EM. Is there a role for preference assessments in research on quality of life in oncology? *Quality of Life Res* 1992;**1**:31–40.
14 Silverman WA, Altman DG. Patients' preferences and randomised trials. *Lancet* 1996;**347**:171–4.
15 Zelen M. A new design for randomized clinical trials. *N Engl J Med* 1979;**300**: 1242–5.
16 Olschewski M, Scheurlen H. Comprehensive cohort study: An alternative to randomized consent design in a breast preservation trial. *Methods Inform Med* 1985;**24**:131–4.
17 Brewin CR, Bradley C. Patient preferences and randomised clinical trials. *BMJ* 1989;**299**:684–5.
18 Paradise JL, Bluestone CD, Rogers KD, Taylor FH, Colborn DK, Bachman RZ, Bernard BS, Schwarzbach RH. Efficacy of adenoidectomy for recurrent

otitis media in children previously treated with tympanostomy-tube placement: Results of parallel randomized and nonrandomized trials. *JAMA* 1990;**263**: 2066–73.

19 Torgerson DJ, Klaber-Moffett J, Russell IT. Patient preferences in randomised trials: threat or opportunity? *J Health Services Res Policy* 1996;**1**:194–7.

3 Bias in RCTs: beyond the sequence generation

The main appeal of the randomised controlled trial (RCT) in health care derives from its potential for reducing selection bias. As discussed in Chapter 1, researchers expect that randomisation, if done properly, can keep study groups as similar as possible at the outset, thus enabling the investigators to isolate and quantify the effect of the interventions they are studying and control for other factors. No other study design allows researchers to balance unknown prognostic factors at baseline. Random allocation does not, however, protect RCTs against other types of bias.

During the past 10 years, important, albeit isolated, research efforts have used RCTs as the subject rather than the tool of research. These studies are usually designed to generate empirical evidence to improve the design, reporting, dissemination, and use of RCTs in health care.[1] These studies have shown that RCTs are vulnerable to multiple types of bias at all stages of their lifespan. Random allocation of the participants to different study groups only increases the potential of a study to be free of bias. Therefore, as a reader, you must be aware that most RCTs are at risk of bias and that bias can arise from many sources, including yourself. It is against this background that I would like to devote this chapter to the concept of bias, highlighting its main sources and sharing with you some strategies that could help you identify it and minimise its impact on your decisions.

What is bias?

In the lay literature, bias has been defined as "opinion or feeling that strongly favours one side in an argument or one item in a group or series; predisposition; prejudice".[2] In health care research, however, bias is defined as any factor or process that tends to deviate the results or conclusions of a trial systematically away from the truth.[3-6] This deviation from the truth can result in underestimation or exaggeration of the effects of an intervention. As there is usually more interest in showing that a new intervention works than in showing that it does not work or that it is harmful, bias in clinical trials usually leads to an exaggeration in the magnitude or importance of the effects of new interventions. Unlike the lay meaning of bias, bias in health research should not be associated immediately with a malicious attempt of investigators, funders, or readers to bend the results of a trial. Although bias can be introduced into a trial voluntarily, it is probably involuntary in most cases.

Bias can occur in a trial during the planning stages, the selection of participants, the administration of interventions, the measurement of outcomes, the analysis of data, the interpretation and reporting of results, and the publication of reports.[3] Bias can also occur when a person is reading the report of a trial.[4]

How can you tell that bias is present in an RCT?

The main reason to anticipate, detect, quantify, and control bias is that the true effects of any health care intervention are unknown. In fact, the whole purpose of RCTs, as well as any other study or research enquiry, is to produce results from a sample of participants that could be generalised to the target population at large. It is impossible ever to know for sure whether the results of a study are biased, simply because it is impossible to establish whether such results depart systematically from a truth that is unknown. Despite this major limitation, many possible sources of biases have been recognised over the years. The existence of most of these biases is supported mainly by common sense. Few studies have been designed specifically to generate empirical data to support the existence of different types of bias and to quantify them. This remains at the same time one of the most exciting and important areas of methodological research, and one of the most neglected.[3]

In this chapter I focus on biases that relate directly to RCTs and bring to your attention any empirical methodological studies that support their existence.

What are the main types of bias in RCTs?

Traditionally, discussions on bias focus on biases that can occur at any point during the course of a trial, from the allocation of participants to study groups, through the delivery of interventions and the measurement of outcomes, to the interpretation and

29

reporting of results. Other types of bias that tend to receive less attention can also, however, have a profound influence on the way in which the results of RCTs are interpreted and used. These biases can occur during the dissemination of a trial from the investigators to potential users, or during the uptake of trial information by potential users of the trial.

To illustrate how bias can affect the results of an RCT, I would like to invite you to focus on the following hypothetical scenario:

Imagine a new drug for the treatment of multiple sclerosis, which has shown promising results in animal studies and in phase I trials. These results, which suggest that the drug can delay the onset of severe motor compromise, have been widely publicised by the media during the past three months. As a result of these results, patient advocacy groups are putting pressure on the Government to make the new drug available as soon as possible. As multiple sclerosis is a debilitating disease that affects millions of people world wide and for which there is no known cure, the investigators (all clinicians who have dealt with multiple sclerosis patients for years), the company producing the new drug (which has invested millions in developing the drug), the media (interested in confirming the results that they so widely publicised), and the potential participants (patients with multiple sclerosis who have been waiting for an effective treatment to be discovered) are all interested in finding the new compound effective. After many intense sessions debating the course of action, a multidisciplinary task force created by the Government, including consumer representatives, agrees that the next step should be a randomised clinical trial. A research protocol is produced by another multidisciplinary panel of investigators and consumers, and a well known research group at a large health care centre is selected to conduct the study.

Elements of this hypothetical scenario will be discussed in the sections that follow.

What biases can occur during the course of a trial?

Selection bias

Selection bias occurs when the outcomes of a trial are affected by systematic differences in the way in which individuals are accepted or rejected for a trial, or in the way in which the interventions are assigned to individuals once they have been accepted into a trial. Prevention of this type of bias is the main justification for the use of RCTs to compare and evaluate different interventions in health care. With true randomisation, all the study participants are given the same opportunity to be allocated or assigned to each of the study groups. In other words, if a trial is truly randomised, group allocation cannot be influenced by the investigators or the study participants.

A perfectly randomised method to allocate participants to the study groups does not, however, protect an RCT from selection bias. Selection bias can be introduced if some potentially eligible individuals are selectively excluded from the study because of prior knowledge of the group to which they would be allocated if they participated in the study. Imagine that the investigator in charge of recruiting patients for the multiple sclerosis trial thinks that depressed patients are less likely to respond to the new drug. The trial is not designed to detect depression in the participants and he is the only person with access to the allocation sequence (which has been generated by computer and is locked in his desk). This investigator could introduce bias into the trial, knowingly or unknowingly, just by making it more difficult for depressive patients to receive the new drug. He can achieve this in at least two ways: first, he can make depressive patients allocated to receive the new drug fit exclusion criteria more easily and more frequently than if they had been allocated to the placebo group; second, he can present information on the trial to depressive patients allocated to receive the new drug in such a way that they would be discouraged from giving consent to participate in the trial. At the end of the trial, if the investigator was right, and depressive patients were less likely to respond to the new drug, the trial will show an exaggerated effect of the new drug during the treatment of multiple sclerosis, as a result of the disproportionate number of depressive patients in the placebo group.

There is empirical evidence confirming that the effects of new interventions can be exaggerated if the randomisation sequence is not concealed from the investigators at the time of obtaining consent from prospective trial participants.[7,8] One study showed that trials with inadequate allocation concealment can exaggerate the effects of interventions by as much as 40% on average.[8] The irony is that allocation concealment is a very simple manoeuvre which can be incorporated into the design of any trial and which can always be implemented.

Despite its simplicity as a manoeuvre and its importance in reducing bias, allocation concealment is rarely reported and perhaps rarely implemented in RCTs. A recent study showed that allocation concealment was reported in less than 10% of articles describing RCTs published in prominent journals in five different languages.[9] This does not mean necessarily that allocation is not concealed in 90% of RCTs. In some cases allocation may have been concealed, but the authors, peer-reviewers, and journal editors were not aware of how important it was to mention it (it takes about a line in the report of an RCT, so "space limitation" is not a good excuse!). If, however, in most cases in which allocation concealment has not been reported, it has not been done, then the majority of RCTs are at risk of exaggerating the effects of the interventions they were designed to evaluate.

Even if the report of an RCT states that efforts were made to conceal the allocation sequence, there are many ways in which randomisation can be subverted by investigators who want to break the allocation code before they obtain consent from prospective trial participants.[10] Even when the allocation codes are kept in sealed opaque envelopes, investigators, for instance, can look through the envelopes using powerful lights or even open the envelope using steam and reseal it without others noticing.[10]

The corollary is that it is very easy to introduce selection bias in RCTs and that readers should not get a false sense of security from a description of a study as randomised. Perhaps the only way to help RCTs achieve what they have set out to achieve is through intensive educational campaigns to increase awareness among investigators, peer-reviewers, journal editors, and users about the importance of adequate randomisation, adequate allocation concealment, and adequate reporting of both.

Ascertainment bias

Ascertainment bias occurs when the results or conclusions of a trial are systematically distorted by knowledge of which intervention each participant is receiving. Ascertainment bias can be introduced by the person administering the interventions, the person receiving the interventions (the participants), the investigator assessing or analysing the outcomes, and even by the people who write the report describing the trial.

The best way to protect a trial against ascertainment bias is by keeping the people involved in the trial unaware of the identity of the interventions for as long as possible. This is also called blinding or masking. The strategies that can be used to reduce ascertainment bias can be applied during at least two periods of a trial. The first period includes the time during which data are collected actively, from the administration of the interventions to the gathering of outcome data. The second period occurs after data have been collected, from data analysis to the reporting of results.

It is important that you recognise the difference between biases that are the result of lack of allocation concealment and biases that arise from lack of blinding. Allocation concealment helps to prevent selection bias, protects the randomisation sequence *before and until the interventions are given to study participants*, and can always be implemented.[8] Blinding helps prevent ascertainment bias, protects the randomisation sequence *after allocation*, and cannot always be implemented.[8]

How can ascertainment bias be reduced during data collection?
Ascertainment bias can be introduced in different ways during data collection. For instance, the people administering the interventions can bias the results of a trial by altering systematically the co-interventions given to participants during the trial. Following our example of the multiple sclerosis trial, the new drug may appear to be more effective at the end of the trial if patients allocated to the new drug received physiotherapy earlier and more intensively than patients allocated to placebo. If participants know that they have been allocated to the placebo group, they are likely to feel disappointed and less willing to report improvement at each of the study time-points. In addition, if the people in charge of assessing and recording the outcomes know which patients are allocated to each of the study groups, they could, consciously or unconsciously, tend to record the outcomes for patients receiving the new drug in a more favourable way than for patients receiving placebo.

In ideal circumstances, ascertainment bias should be reduced by blinding the individuals who administer the interventions, the participants who receive the interventions, and the individuals in charge of assessing and recording the outcomes. In most cases, the interventions are either administered and assessed by the same group of investigators, or self administered by the study participants. Therefore, the degree of blinding required to reduce ascertainment bias during data collection is usually achieved by double-blind trials (see Chapter 2).

The importance of blinding has been confirmed in empirical studies. It has been shown, for instance, that open studies are more likely to favour experimental interventions over the controls[11] and that studies that are not double-blinded can exaggerate effect estimates by 17%.[8] Despite the empirical evidence available, and common sense, it has been shown recently that only about half of the trials that could be double-blinded actually achieved double-blinding.[12] Even when the trials are described as double-blind, most reports do not provide adequate information on how blinding was achieved or statements on the perceived success (or failure) of double-blinding efforts.[12–14]

The best strategy to achieve blinding during data collection is with the use of placebos. Placebos are inert substances that are intended to be indistinguishable from the active interventions. To be successful, placebos should be identical to the active interventions in all aspects, except for the components of the active intervention that have specific and predictable mechanisms of action. Placebos do not apply only to trials evaluating pharmacological interventions. They also apply to non-drug interventions such as psychological, physical, and surgical interventions. Placebos are certainly easier to develop and implement successfully in drug trials. In these cases they should resemble the taste, smell, and colour of the active drug, and should be given using an identical procedure.

Placebos are more difficult to develop and implement successfully in non-drug trials. For example, it is difficult to develop and implement placebo counselling, physiotherapy, acupuncture, or electrical stimulation. In some cases it is impossible, unfeasible, or simply unethical to use placebos. It would be impossible, for example, to use a placebo intervention in a trial evaluating the effect on mothers and newborns of early versus late discharge from hospital after childbirth. On the other hand, it would be unfeasible or unethical to use a placebo in trials evaluating new or existing surgical interventions (although there are examples of trials in which placebo surgery has been used successfully to challenge the perceived effectiveness of established surgical interventions). In addition, there is controversy as to whether placebo-controlled studies are ethical to study a new or existing intervention when there is an effective intervention available. Even in cases where the use of placebos is impossible, unfeasible, or unethical, trials can be at least single-blind. In a surgical or acupuncture trial, for instance, single-blinding can be achieved by keeping the investigators in charge of assessing the outcomes unaware of which participants receive which interventions.

How can ascertainment bias be reduced after data collection?
Ascertainment bias can be introduced easily after data collection, if the investigators in charge of analysing or reporting the results of the trial are aware of which participants are receiving which interventions. The effects of a new intervention can be enhanced, for instance, if the investigators in charge of analysing the trial data select the outcomes and the time-points that show maximum benefit from the new intervention, and ignore outcomes and time-points that show either no effect or harm from the new intervention. Similarly, investigators in charge of reporting the trial results can choose to emphasise the outcomes and time-points that show the maximum effects of the new intervention, downplaying or ignoring findings which suggest that the new intervention is equivalent to or less effective than the control.

This source of bias can be controlled by keeping the data analysts and the people in charge of reporting the trial results unaware of the identity of the study groups. In a study with two groups, for instance, the outcome data could be given to analysts coded as A and B and, once they complete the analysis, the results could be given to the person in charge of writing the report using the same codes. The codes would not be broken until after the data analysis and reporting phases were completed. These strategies are rarely used.

The frequency and magnitude of ascertainment bias introduced after data collection have not been studied at all.

Other biases that can be introduced during the course of a trial

Bias introduced by inappropriate handling of withdrawals, drop outs, and protocol violations   Ideally, all participants in a trial should complete the study, follow the protocol, and provide data on all the outcomes of interest at all time-points. In reality, however, most trials have missing data. Data can be missing because some of the participants drop out before the end of the trial, because participants do not follow the protocol either deliberately or accidentally, or because some outcomes are not measured correctly or cannot be measured at all at one or more time-points. Regardless of the cause, inappropriate handling of the missing information can lead to bias. For instance, if in the multiple sclerosis trial patients who do not obtain benefit from the new drug withdraw more frequently because of adverse effects, their exclusion from analysis would lead the investigators to exaggerate the benefit and underestimate the harm of the new drug. This bias can occur independently of whether or not the investigators are aware of the identity of the interventions received by the participants when they are considering withdrawal of some participants from the study. If the decisions on withdrawals have been made because of knowledge of the interventions received by the participants, this constitutes yet another cause of ascertainment bias.

On occasion, however, it is impossible to know the status of participants at the times when the missing information should have been collected. This could happen, for example, if participants move to different areas during the study or fail to contact the investigators for an unknown reason. Excluding these participants or specific outcome measurements from the final analysis can also lead to bias.

The only strategy that can confidently be assumed to eliminate bias in these circumstances includes two components. The first is called "intention to treat" analysis, and means that all the study participants are included in the analyses as part of the groups to which they were randomised regardless of whether they completed the study or not. The second component includes a "worst case scenario" sensitivity analysis. This is performed by assigning the worst possible outcomes to the missing patients or time-points in the group that shows the best results, and the best possible outcomes to the missing patients or time-points in the group with the worst results, and evaluating whether the new analysis contradicts or supports the results of the initial analysis which does not take into account the missing data.

Bias introduced by inappropriate use of cross-over design It is important that certain criteria are met when deciding whether a crossover design is appropriate to answer a particular research question. The most important criterion is that cross-over trials should not be used for the study of curable or lethal conditions. A clear description of the other criteria, and the advantages and disadvantages of cross-over trials, are described in Chapter 2.

What biases can occur during dissemination of the trials?

The main sources of bias during dissemination of trials are publication bias, language bias, country of publication bias, time lag bias, and potential breakthrough bias.

What is publication bias?

Some evidence shows a propensity for investigators and sponsors to write and submit, and for peer-reviewers and editors to accept, manuscripts for publication depending on the direction of the findings. This tendency, which appears to favour trials with positive results, has been called publication bias.[15–17] A systematic review of five empirical methodological studies published mostly during the past 10 years confirmed that the failure to publish is not a random event, but is heavily influenced by the direction and strength of research findings, whereby manuscripts with statistically significant ("positive") results are published preferentially over manuscripts reporting non-significant ("negative") results.[17] Publication bias may be the main factor behind the systematic differences found between studies funded by industry and their counterparts.[18]

The only way to eliminate publication bias is through compulsory registration of trials at inception and publication of the results of all trials. Although highly desirable, compulsory registration of trials and publication of the results of all trials are the focus of intense debate and controversy fuelled by strong ethical and economic elements, and are unlikely to happen in the near future. Until they happen, readers must be aware that, by relying on published studies to guide their decisions, they are always at risk of overestimating the effect of interventions.

What is language bias?

Recently, a variation of publication bias has been described as "language bias", to indicate that manuscripts may be submitted to and published by journals in different languages depending on the direction of their results, with more studies with positive results published in English.[19]

What is country of publication bias?

It has also been shown that researchers in some countries may publish only positive results, such as with RCTs evaluating acupuncture conducted in China, Japan, Hong Kong, and Taiwan.[20]

What is time lag bias?

This bias occurs when the speed of publication depends on the direction and strength of the trial results.[1] In general, it seems that trials with "negative" results take twice as long to be published as "positive" trials. Studies on this type of bias also show that trials may take years to be submitted and published after completion; that the time taken to complete trials is similar to the time it then takes to publish them; and that large trials take as long as small trials to be published.[21,22]

What is "potential breakthrough" bias?

This type of bias can be introduced by journalists (and, increasingly, Internet publishers) if they systematically select, overrate, and disseminate trials depending on the direction of the findings. This could occur, for instance, when journalists bring to public attention the results of a trial purporting beneficial effects of a new intervention for an incurable disease, while they ignore the results of previous (or concurrent) trials in which the same intervention showed no benefit.[23] This media coverage may influence the decisions of clinicians and patients who are not aware of the other studies. This type of bias is closely related to a group of biases that occur during the uptake of information and which will be discussed in the next section.

What biases can occur during the uptake of information by users?

More than 15 years ago, different types of reader biases were described.[4] At the time in which they were reported, the existence of these biases was supported only by common sense and experience. Recently, there have been empirical studies that support the existence of reader bias, showing that there are systematic differences in the way readers assess the quality of RCTs, depending on whether the assessments are conducted under masked or open conditions.[13,24] These studies do not, however, focus on any specific type of reader bias. More research is needed to establish the individual contribution of each type of reader bias.

The following is a description of the reader biases described by Owen[4] with a few more added by myself.

Rivalry bias Underrating the strengths or exaggerating the weaknesses of studies published by a rival.

"I owe him one" bias This is a variation of the previous bias and occurs when a reader (particularly a peer-reviewer) accepts flawed results from a study by someone who did the same for the reader.

Personal habit bias Overrating or underrating a study depending on the habits of the reader (for example, a reader who enjoys eating animal fat overrating a study that challenges the adverse effects of animal fat on health).

Moral bias Overrating or underrating a study depending on how much it agrees or disagrees with the reader's morals (for example, a reader who regards abortion as immoral overrating a study showing a relationship between abortion and breast cancer).

Clinical practice bias Overrating or underrating a study according to whether the study supports or challenges the reader's current or past clinical practice (that is, a clinician who gives lidocaine to patients with acute myocardial infarction, underrating a study which suggests that lidocaine may increase mortality in these patients).

Territory bias This is related to the previous bias and can occur when readers overrate studies that support their own specialty or profession (for example, a surgeon favouring a study which suggests that surgery is more effective than medical treatment, or obstetricians underrating a study which suggests that midwives can provide adequate care during uncomplicated pregnancies and deliveries).

Complementary medicine bias I have added this to Owen's list. It refers to the systematic overrating or underrating of studies that describe complementary medicine interventions, particularly when the results suggest that the interventions are effective.

"Do something" bias   Overrating a study which suggests that an intervention is effective, particularly when there is no effective intervention available. This is a bias that may be common among clinicians and patients (for example, a patient with AIDS overrating a study describing a cure for AIDS).

"Do nothing" bias   This bias is related to the previous one. It occurs when readers underrate a study that discourages the use of an intervention in conditions for which no effective treatment exists. This bias may be common among researchers and academics (that is, a researcher underrating a study which shows that membrane stabilisers do not provide analgesia in patients with painful diabetic neuropathy unresponsive to any other treatment).

Favoured design bias   Overrating a study that uses a design supported, publicly or privately, by the reader (for example, a consumer advocate overrating an RCT that takes into account patient preferences).

Disfavoured design bias   The converse of favoured design bias. It occurs when a study is underrated because it uses a design that is not favoured by the reader (for example, a reader underrating a crossover trial, even when it meets all the criteria described in Chapter 2).

Resource allocation bias   Overrating or underrating a study according to the reader's preference for resource allocation. This bias may be one of the most frequently found in health care, because it can emanate from consumers, clinicians, policy makers, researchers, and fund holders.

Prestigious journal bias   This occurs when the results of studies published in prestigious journals are overrated.

Non-prestigious journal bias   The converse of prestigious journal bias. It occurs when the results of studies published in non-prestigious journals are underrated.

Printed word bias   This occurs when a study is overrated because of undue confidence in published data.

"Lack-of-peer-review" bias I have added this one to Owen's list. It occurs when a reader underrates a study, published or unpublished, because it has not been peer-reviewed.

Prominent author bias This occurs when the results of studies published by prominent authors are overrated.

Unknown or non-prominent author bias Owen called this the "who is he?" bias. It occurs when the results of studies published by unknown or non-prominent authors are underrated.

Famous institution bias This occurs when the results of studies emanating from famous institutions are overrated.

Unrecognised or non-prestigious institution bias Related to the previous bias. It occurs when the results of studies emanating from unrecognised or non-prestigious institutions are systematically underrated.

Large trial bias I have added this to Owen's list. It occurs when the results of large trials are overrated.

Multicentre trial bias I have added this to Owen's list. It occurs when the results of multicentre collaborative trials are overrated. These trials do not necessarily have large sample sizes.

Small trial bias I have also added this to Owen's list. It occurs when the results of trials with small sample size are underrated, particularly when they contradict the opinion of the reader (that is, attributing to chance any statistically or clinically significant effect found by a small trial, or any lack of significant effects to low power).

"Flashy title" bias It occurs when the results of studies with attractive titles are overrated (particularly by patients or journalists) or underrated (particularly by academics, if they regard them as sensationalist!).

Substituted question bias It occurs when a reader substitutes a question for the question that the study is designed to answer, and

41

regards the results of the study as invalid if they do not answer the substituted question.

Credential or professional background bias Overrating or underrating the results of a study according to the qualifications of the authors (for example, physicians underrating research done by nurses or vice versa; basic scientists underrating research done by clinicians or vice versa; PhDs underrating studies published by MDs and vice versa; readers overrating research by authors with many letters after their names and vice versa).

Esteemed author bias Includes Owen's "esteemed professor bias" and the "friendship bias". This bias occurs when the reader overrates results obtained by a close friend or mentor.

Geography bias This occurs when studies are overrated or underrated according to the country or region where it was conducted.

Language bias of publication Overrating or underrating a study depending on the language in which it is reported (that is, the belief that studies published in languages other than English are of inferior quality to those published in English).

Omission bias This occurs when a study is overrated or underrated because the reader did not read a key section.

Tradition bias Overrating or underrating the results of a study depending on whether it supports or challenges traditional procedures (that is, underrating a study that challenges episiotomy during normal vaginal deliveries).

Bankbook bias Overrating or underrating a study depending on the impact of its results on the income of the reader (for example, a surgeon underrating a study that questions the need for surgery to relieve back pain in patients with spinal stenosis, or a pharmaceutical company overrating the results of a study that supports the use of one of its products).

Belligerence bias Underrating studies systematically just for the sake of being difficult.

Technology bias Overrating (Owen's pro-technology bias) or underrating (Owen's anti-technology bias) a study according to the reader's attraction to or aversion for technology in health care.

Empiricism bias Overrating or underrating a study because it challenges the clinical experience of the reader.

"I am an epidemiologist bias" This occurs when the reader repudiates a study that contains any flaw, albeit minor, in its design, analysis, or interpretation.

1 Jadad AR, Rennie D. The randomized controlled trial gets a middle-aged checkup. *JAMA* 1998;**279**:319–20.
2 Hornby AS. *Oxford advanced learner's dictionary of current English*, 4th edn. Oxford: Oxford University Press, 1989.
3 Sackett DL. Bias in analytic research. *J Chronic Dis* 1979;**32**:51–63.
4 Owen R. Reader bias. *JAMA* 1982;**247**:2533–4.
5 Andersen B. *Methodological errors in medical research*. Oxford: Blackwell Scientific, 1990.
6 Fletcher RH, Fletcher SW, Wagner EH. *Clinical epidemiology: the essentials*, 3rd edn. Baltimore, MD: Williams & Wilkins, 1996.
7 Chalmers TC, Celano P, Sacks HS, Smith H. Bias in treatment assignment in controlled clinical trials. *N Engl J Med* 1983;**309**:1359–61.
8 Schulz KF, Chalmers I, Hayes RJ, Altman DG. Empirical evidence of bias: dimensions of methodological quality associated with estimates of treatment effects in controlled trials. *JAMA* 1995;**273**:408–12.
9 Moher D, Fortin P, Jadad AR, Juni P, Klassen T, Le Lorier J, Liberati A, Linde K, Penna A. Completeness of reporting of trials published in languages other than English: implications for conduct and reporting of systematic reviews. *Lancet* 1996;**347**:363–6.
10 Schulz KF. Subverting randomization in controlled trials. *JAMA* 1995;**274**: 1456–8.
11 Colditz GA, Miller JN, Mosteller F. How study design affects outcomes in comparisons of therapy. I. Therapy. *Stat Med* 1989;**8**:441–54.
12 Schulz KF, Grimes DA, Altman DG, Hayes RJ. Blinding and exclusions after allocation in randomised controlled trials: survey of published parallel group trials in obstetrics and gynaecology. *BMJ* 1996;**312**:742–4.
13 Jadad AR, Moore RA, Carroll D, Jenkinson C, Reynolds JM, Gavaghan DJ, McQuay DM. Assessing the quality of reports on randomized clinical trials: Is blinding necessary? *Controlled Clin Trials* 1996;**17**:1–12.
14 Moher D, Jadad AR, Tugwell P. Assessing the quality of randomized controlled trials. *Int J Technol Assess Health Care* 1996;**12**:195–208.
15 Dickersin K. The existence of publication bias and risk factors for its occurrence. *JAMA* 1990;**263**:1385–9.
16 Rennie D, Flanagin A. Publication bias—the triumph of hope over experience. *JAMA* 1992;**267**:411–12.
17 Dickersin K. How important is publication bias? A synthesis of available data. *AIDS Educ Prev* 1997;**9**(suppl A):15–21.

18 Bero LA, Rennie D. Influences on the quality of published drug trials. *Int J Technol Assess Health Care* 1996;**12**:209–37.

19 Egger M, Zellweger-Zahner T, Schneider M, Junker C, Lengeler C, Antes G. Language bias in randomised controlled trials published in English and German. *Lancet* 1997;**350**:326–9.

20 Vickers A, Goyal N, Harland R, Rees R. Do certain countries produce only positive results? A systematic review of controlled trials. *Controlled Clin Trials* 1998; **19**:159–66.

21 Ioannidis JPA. Effect of the statistical significance of results on the time to completion and publication of randomized efficacy trials: a survival analysis. *JAMA* 1998;**279**:281–6.

22 Stern JM, Simes RJ. Publication bias: evidence of delayed publication in a cohort study of clinical research projects. *BMJ* 1997;**315**:640–5.

23 Koren G, Klein N. Bias against negative studies in newspaper reports of medical research. *JAMA* 1991;**266**:1824–6.

24 McNutt RA, Evans AT, Fletcher RH, Fletcher SW. The effects of blinding on the quality of peer-review. A randomized trial. *JAMA* 1990;**263**:1371–6.

4 Assessing the quality of RCTs: why, what, how, and by whom?

If all trials were perfect, you would not have to worry about their quality. Instead, you could always use them with confidence as part of your decisions. To be perfect, among other things, trials would have to do the following:

- Answer clear and relevant clinical questions previously unanswered.
- Evaluate all possible interventions for all possible variations of the conditions of interest, in all possible types of patients, in all settings, using all relevant outcome measures.
- Include all available patients.
- Include strategies to eliminate bias during the administration of the interventions, the evaluation of the outcomes, and reporting of the results, thus reflecting the true effect of the interventions.
- Include perfect statistical analyses.
- Be described in reports written in clear and unambiguous language, including an exact account of all the events that occurred during the design and course of the trial, as well as individual patient data, and an accurate description of the patients who were included, excluded, withdrawn, and dropped out.
- Be designed, conducted, and reported by researchers who did not have conflicts of interest.
- Follow strict ethical principles.

Unfortunately, there is no such as thing as a perfect trial. In real life, readers only have imperfect trials to read and face lots of barriers to determining their quality with confidence.

One of the main barriers that hinders the formal assessment of trial quality is that quality is a complex concept or "construct". As with any other construct, such as anxiety, happiness, or love, quality can be acknowledged without difficulty, but it is not easy to define or measure.

Another major barrier is that there is an increasing number of tools available to assess trial quality, but little empirical evidence to guide the selection of tools and the incorporation of assessments into reviews and decisions. There is also little empirical evidence about who should do the assessments (number and background of assessors), about how the assessments should be done (that is, masked vs open conditions), or about the impact of the assessments on health care decisions.

A third major barrier hindering the assessment of trial quality is that, in most cases, the only way to assess quality is by relying on information contained in the written report. The problem is that a trial with a biased design that is well reported could be judged as having high quality, whereas a well designed but poorly reported trial could be judged as having low quality.

In this chapter, I discuss each of these barriers, present the results of recent empirical methodological studies that could help you overcome them, discuss recent efforts to improve the quality of reports of RCTs, and identify areas where further methodological research is required. I hope that the information you find in this chapter will help you not only if you are a clinician trying to decide whether to include an intervention in your armamentarium, but also if you are reading a systematic review and want to evaluate the effect that the assessment of trial quality may have had on the results of the review (see Chapter 7).

Regardless of why you want to assess the quality of a trial or group of trials, the first question that you should try to answer is: What is quality?

What is quality?

Quality means different things to different people. Specific aspects of trials that have been used to define and assess trial quality include the following:[1,2]

- The clinical relevance of the research question.
- The internal validity of the trial (the degree to which the trial design, conduct, analysis, and presentation have minimised or avoided biased comparisons of the interventions under evaluation).
- The external validity (the precision and extent to which it is possible to generalise the results of the trial to other settings).
- The appropriateness of data analysis and presentation.

- The ethical implications of the intervention they evaluate.

You could define quality by focusing on a single aspect of trials or on a combination of any of the above.[1,2] You should, however, take into account that the relevance of the research question, the degree of generalisability of the results, the adequacy of data analysis and presentation, and the ethical implications depend on the context in which they are assessed (that is, they are very much in the eye of the beholder). Of all the aspects of a trial that have been used to define and assess quality, internal validity is the least context-dependent and perhaps the only one that has been the subject of the few empirical methodological studies available. As a result of this, I would recommend that you always include elements related to internal validity in any assessment of the trial quality, complementing them with other aspects of the trial that may be relevant to your specific circumstances. Consider, for example, a trial in which a new antidepressant has been studied in affluent men with suicidal ideation and shown to reduce suicide rates. The generalisability of the results of this trial would be very important if you were a clinician trying to decide whether to offer it to an indigent woman, but would be irrelevant if you were a peer-reviewer trying to decide whether to recommend the report for publication. The internal validity of the trial would, however, be important in both cases. Internal validity is an important and necessary component of the assessment of trial quality, but it is not sufficient to provide a comprehensive evaluation of a trial.

What type of tools can be used to assess trial quality?

Once you establish what quality means to you, the next step is to select a tool to generate the assessments. At this point you can develop your own tool or you can use an existing one.

What is involved in developing a new tool to assess trial quality?

If you decide to develop your own tool, you can create the tool by selecting a single item or a group of items that you (and perhaps a group of colleagues) regard as important according to your definition of quality, decide how to score each item, and use the tool straight away. For example, after deciding to focus on internal

47

and external validity, you could select "concealment of allocation" as the only item for judging internal validity, and "definition of inclusion and exclusion criteria" and "description of the primary outcome" as markers of external validity. After selecting the items, you can decide, on your own or after discussion with your colleagues, to assign two points to a trial with adequate concealment and one point each for adequate descriptions of inclusion/exclusion criteria and the primary outcome. Once you have the items and the scoring system, you can just apply them to trials and obtain scores that would reflect their quality. The advantage of this approach is that it is relatively simple and always yields an assessment tool. The disadvantage is that tools created using this informal approach can produce variable assessments of the same trials when used by multiple individuals, and may not be able to discriminate between studies with good and poor quality.

Alternatively, you could develop the new tool following established methodological procedures similar to those used in the formal development of any other type of health measurement tool. The advantages of this approach are that it is systematic, it can be replicated by others (if properly described), and it can yield tools with known reliability and construct validity which would allow readers to discriminate among trials of varied quality. A description of these procedures is beyond the scope of this book, but can be found elsewhere.[3] The following is, however, a list of the steps for developing a new tool to assess trial quality:

- Definition of the construct "quality" (as described in the previous section).
- Definition of the scope of the tool: for instance, the tool could be condition specific (that is, assess only the quality of trials in obstetrics) or intervention specific (that is, assess trials evaluating different types of episiotomies).
- Definition of the population of end users: the tool could be designed for use by clinicians, statisticians or patients, or by individuals with any background.
- Selection of candidate items to include in the tool: usually, this is achieved by asking a group of individuals to propose items to include in the tool, selecting them from items in existing tools, or using their own judgment and expertise.
- Development of a prototype tool: this is usually achieved by getting the individuals who proposed items to meet and decide,

by consensus, on the essential group of items that should be included in the tool. At this point, the group can also decide on the wording of each item and on a scoring system. The prototype could be tested by using it to score a small group of trials and, using the experience gathered during the process, to refine the wording and modify the order in which the items are presented.

- Selection of targets: once a prototype tool has been developed, the developers should select a group of trials to be assessed using the tool. These trials have different judged degrees of quality (that is, some should be regarded as having poor quality, whereas others should be regarded as having high quality).

- Selection of raters: the developers should select a group of individuals to use the tool to score the target trials. The characteristics of these individuals should reflect the potential users of the tool.

- Assessment of the trials: the trials are given to the raters to assess, with or without previous training on the use of the tool.

- Evaluation of the consistency of the assessments: this involves measurement of the degree to which different raters agree on the quality of the trials. This is called interobserver or interrater reliability. Reliability is also referred to as consistency or agreement. Rarely, this also includes an evaluation of the degree of intraobserver or intrarater reliability, or the degree of agreement between quality assessments done by the same raters on separate occasions. There are several methods to measure the consistency of the measurements (for example, percentage agreement, κ, correlation coefficient, intraclass correlation coefficient). A description of these methods and their advantages and limitations is described elsewhere.[3]

- Evaluation of "construct" validity: in this case, validity refers to the ability of the tool to measure what it is believed to be measuring. One important limitation to the evaluation of the construct validity of a tool for assessing trial quality is the lack of a gold standard. To overcome this limitation, the developers usually have to make predictions on how the tool would rate trials previously judged as having different quality and testing these predictions. In this case, you would expect the tool to differentiate between the trials previously judged as having poor quality and those judged as having good quality.

- Proposal of a refined tool: once the tool is shown to be reliable and valid, it is ready for use.

The main disadvantage of developing a new tool is that it is a time-consuming process. To avoid developing a new tool using the established methodology or creating one without proper evaluation, the reader can choose to select an existing tool.

How many tools exist to evaluate trial quality?

Existing tools to assess trial quality can be classified broadly into those that include individual components and those that include groups of components.

A component represents an item that describes a single aspect of quality. Assessing trial quality using a component can be achieved by scoring the component as present or absent or by judging the adequacy of the information available on the component. For example, concealment of patient assignment could be judged as present or absent or, if it could be judged as adequate, unclear or inadequate.[4] There are empirical methodological studies suggesting a relationship between at least five specific components and the likelihood of bias in trials. Most of these studies are described in Chapter 3. Briefly, these studies suggest that trials with inadequate randomisation or double-blinding, inadequate or unclear concealment of allocation, or inappropriately used crossover designs are more likely to produce larger treatment effects than those obtained by their counterparts.[4-7] There is also evidence suggesting that reports of trials sponsored by pharmaceutical companies are more likely to favour the experimental intervention over controls than trials not sponsored by pharmaceutical companies.[8] Even though individual components are quick and easy to score, using a single component to assess quality is not recommended because it provides minimal information about the overall quality of trials.[2]

The narrow view provided by individual components can be overcome by using several components grouped in checklists or scales. The main difference between a checklist and a scale is that, in a checklist, the components are evaluated separately and do not have numerical scores attached to them, whereas, in a scale, each item is scored numerically and an overall quality score is generated.[2] A systematic search of the literature identified nine checklists and 25 scales for assessing trial quality.[9] Ongoing efforts to update this literature search suggest that there are now at least twice as many scales for assessing trial quality and that their number is likely to keep increasing.[10] Among the available checklists and scales, only one has been developed using established methodological procedures.[1]

What are the characteristics of the validated tool to assess trial quality?

The validated tool is a scale (Fig 4.1) that I developed using the steps outlined in the previous sections as part of a doctoral work on pain relief.[11] Since its development, the scale has been used by other investigators who have confirmed that it is easy and quick to use (it takes less than five minutes to score a trial report), provides consistent measurements (even those provided by consumers with no health care background), and has construct validity.[1,9,12–14] The scale has been used successfully to identify systematic differences among trials in the areas of infertility,[7] homoeopathy,[15] anaesthesia,[14] pain relief,[16] and neonatology,[12] as well as in sets of trials published in five different languages.[17,18]

The scale includes three items that are directly related to bias reduction and are presented as questions to elicit "yes" or "no" answers. The scale produces scores from 0 to 5. Point awards for the first two items (randomisation and double-blinding) depend not only on whether the trial is described as randomised or double-blind, but also on the appropriateness of the methods used to

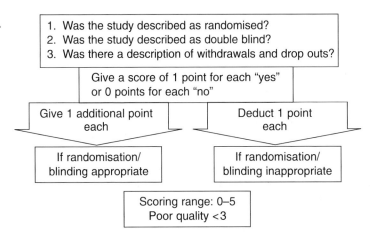

Figure 4.1   Validated quality scale. (From Jadad et al.[1])

randomise and blind the trial. For example, if the trial is described as randomised or double-blind, but there is no description of the methods used to generate the randomisation sequence or the double-blind conditions, 1 point is awarded in each case (that is, 1 point is awarded for randomisation and 1 point for double-blinding if the trial is described as both randomised and double-blind, or only 1 point is awarded if the trial is described as randomised but not as double-blind). If the methods of generating the randomisation sequence or creating blinded conditions are described and are appropriate, 1 additional point is given for each item (see Chapter 3). Conversely, if the methods used to generate the randomisation sequence or create blinded conditions are described, but inappropriate, the relevant item is given 0 points. The third item of the scale, withdrawals and drop outs, is awarded 0 points for a negative answer and 1 point for a positive answer. For a positive answer, the number of withdrawals and drop outs *in each group and the reasons* must be stated in the report. If there were no withdrawals, this should also be stated (Fig 4.1). If a trial provides the number and reasons for withdrawals and drop outs in each group, you, as a reader, could reanalyse the data. At the time of the development of the scale, it was debated whether this item should be scored according to the proportion of withdrawals and drop outs in the trials, but this was considered inappropriate because we do not know precisely when a trial has too many drop outs. Once you have scored all the items of the scale, a trial could be judged as having poor quality if it is awarded 2 points or less. It has been shown that studies that obtain 2 or less points are likely to produce treatment effects which are 35% larger than those produced by trials with 3 or more points.[19]

You can use the overall score produced by the scale or use individual items. The use of the individual items is the most appropriate option if you do not feel comfortable with lumping different aspects of a trial into a single score or when the reports describe trials in areas where double-blinding is not feasible or appropriate (that is, surgical trials). Even trials that cannot be double-blind can, however, still be awarded more than 2 points if they were conducted and reported properly, and thus leave the category of poor trials. Trials could be awarded 3 points if they included a description of appropriate methods to generate the randomisation sequence (2 points) and a detailed account of withdrawals and drop outs (1 point).

This scale by no means represents the only or most appropriate way to assess trial quality, but it is the only validated tool available and appears to produce robust and valid results in an increasing number of empirical methodological studies. This does not mean that the scale should be used in isolation. Instead, you should complement it with separate assessments of any components for which there is empirical evidence of a direct relationship with bias. In addition, you could also add separate assessments of any other component or group of components related to other aspects of trial quality (for example, external validity, quality of data analysis, or presentation, and so on) that you think are important in each case. My current practice, for instance, includes the use of the validated scale together with a separate assessment of concealment of allocation, sources of funding, language of publication, country of publication, and, when applicable, the appropriateness of crossover design.

Who should do the assessments and how?

For more than 10 years it has been suggested that the quality of trial reports should be assessed under masked conditions, that is, without the knowledge of the authors, institutions, sponsorship, publication year and journal, or study results.[5] There are, however, only two published empirical studies addressing this issue.[1,20] One of these studies showed that assessments under masked conditions were more likely to yield lower and more consistent scores than assessments under open conditions.[1] The other study also showed that lower scores were obtained under masked conditions.[20] These results imply that bias could be introduced by assessments under open conditions. There is evidence, however, suggesting that the differences in the scores obtained under open or masked conditions may not be important.[20] Masking the reports would reduce the likelihood of bias marginally, but it would also increase the resources required to conduct the assessments. Given the methodological and financial implications of these findings, and the small amount of empirical evidence available, I would not recommend that you mask the trial reports as a mandatory step during the assessment of their quality.

Another issue that you should take into account is the number and background of the people required to assess the quality of a given trial. Again, if you are a clinician trying to keep up to date, this is not an issue, because you will be the only person assessing the quality of a particular trial at a given point in time. If, however, you are reading a systematic review done by others, you may want to see if the authors provide information on who assessed trial quality. Typically, systematic reviewers ask two individuals (called raters, observers, or assessors) to assess the trials independently. They are given copies of the trial reports, the assessment instrument(s) with instructions, and a form on which to complete the assessments. The purpose of using multiple individuals to assess trial quality is to minimise the number of mistakes (usually caused by oversight while reading the trial report), and the risk of bias during the assessments. Once they have completed the assessments, the raters are invited to meet to discuss their findings and agree on a single quality assessment for each trial. Reaching agreement on trial quality is usually easy, but on occasions it may require a third person to act as arbiter. The degree of agreement between the raters can be quantified using methods previously described (that is, percentage agreement, κ, correlation coefficient, intraclass correlation coefficient). These methods and their advantages and limitations have been described elsewhere.[3] If the raters reach consensus, however, the value of measuring interrater agreement is limited.

How can the quality assessments be used?

Once you have assessed the quality of one or more trials, you should use the assessments to guide your decisions. How you use the assessments, however, will depend on your role, the purpose of the quality assessments, and the number of trials on the same topic that you are evaluating. For example:

- If you are a clinician, you may want to use the assessments to judge whether the results of a trial are credible and applicable to your own patients.
- If you are a peer-reviewer or a journal editor, you may want to use the assessments to decide whether a report should be published.
- If you are a researcher planning a new trial, you may want to use the assessments of similar existing trials to decide whether the new trial is justified or, if justified, to improve its design.

- If you are a reviewer, you may want to use the quality assessments to decide how much each trial should influence the overall analysis of all the evidence available on a particular topic.

There are different approaches to incorporate quality assessments into your decisions. If you are a clinician, a peer-reviewer, or a journal editor, and you are dealing with only one trial, you could set thresholds below which the trial would have limited value to guide your clinical decisions or to be published. For instance, if you are a clinician evaluating a trial in which the main outcomes are subjective, you may decide to use the trial to guide your decisions only if it is double-blind and the authors provide a detailed account of co-interventions. In addition, as a journal editor you may decide not to publish trials in which allocation was not concealed and that do not provide a detailed account of the flow of participants.

The situation is more complicated if you are reading or conducting a review of multiple trials on the same topic. In this case, there are several approaches that could be used to incorporate quality assessments,[2,7,21] but little research evidence has evaluated the impact of any of these methods on the results of the reviews.[2] These approaches include the following.

Tabulation of the quality assessments

The only purpose of this approach is to inform the readers of the review about the quality of the evidence provided by the available trials and to let them judge the credibility of such evidence. A variation of this approach is to display the results of each trial in a figure, sorting them in descending order according to their quality.

Use of quality assessments as thresholds to include or exclude trials from a review

This approach is used frequently, but can produce widely variable results, depending on the instrument and the threshold used.[22]

Use of quality assessments to conduct sensitivity analyses

This approach is used (see Chapter 6) to assess the robustness of the conclusions of a systematic review. It includes several steps: first, the quality of all trials included in the review is assessed; second, all trials are grouped according to their quality (that is, one group with trials of low quality and another with trials of high quality); third, the evidence provided by the trials within each group is synthesised; fourth, the evidence provided by all trials, regardless of their quality, is synthesised; fifth, the results of the evidence synthesis is compared across the groups (the results obtained from trials of low quality are compared with the results produced by trials with high quality, and both are compared with the results of the synthesis of the evidence from all trials). If the results are similar across the groups, you could conclude that the effects of the intervention are robust and you should feel confident with the conclusions that you draw. If the results are different, you will have to seek possible reasons and be cautious about the conclusions that you draw from the available evidence. For example, a sensitivity analysis of nine trials on antioestrogens for the treatment of male infertility showed that low quality studies produced a positive effect with treatment, whereas no benefit was observed with high quality trials. The overall synthesis of all trials suggested a marginal improvement in pregnancy rate (in the spouses, of course) with antioestrogen treatment.[7] These discrepant results helped authors conclude that poor studies were exaggerating the overall estimate of treatment effect and that decisions ignoring the results from studies of high quality could lead to more harm than good. This may be the most appropriate approach to incorporate quality assessments in reviews, given that it does not exclude information, allows the reviewer to assess the robustness of the conclusions, and allows the reader to replicate the analyses if necessary.

Use of quality assessments as the input sequence for cumulative meta-analysis

Meta-analysis refers to the statistical combination of the results of independent studies included in a review with the purpose of producing a quantitative estimate of the overall effect of the interventions under evaluation (see Chapter 6). Typically, data from all relevant trials are combined at once. The reviewers, however, may decide to use a technique called cumulative meta-analysis, which combines the trials sequentially. The quality of the trials could be used as the criterion to decide the order in which the trials are selected for combination. For instance, the first meta-analysis would include the combination of the results from the two trials with the highest quality; the second meta-analysis would include the results of the first three trials with the highest quality; and so on. The purpose of this approach is to allow the reviewer to determine the effect of trial quality on overall estimates of effect. Although attractive, little is known about the value of this approach.

Use of quality assessments to "weight" trials included in meta-analyses

This is perhaps the most aggressive method to incorporate quality assessments in reviews. It requires the incorporation of the actual quality assessments into the conventional formulae used to conduct meta-analysis. The purpose of this approach is to allow trials of high quality to influence the overall effect estimate more than trials with low quality. This is the least studied approach and the most likely to provide estimates that will vary according to the method used to report the quality assessments.

Recent efforts to improve the quality of reporting of RCTs

By this point I hope that you will be convinced that a major barrier hindering the assessment of trial quality is that, in most cases, we must rely on the information contained in the written report. The problem is that a trial with a biased design that is well reported could be judged as having high quality, whereas a well designed but poorly reported trial could be judged as having low quality. If you contact the authors of the report directly, they may be able to provide the missing information that you require to complete the quality assessments, but they may not have such information available or they may give you false information (that is, it would be easy for them to tell you that a trial that they published 20 years ago included concealment of allocation). Ideally, all these problems could be avoided if the authors of trial reports provided enough information for the readers to judge whether the results of the trials are reliable.

In 1996, a group of clinical epidemiologists, biostatisticians, and journal editors published a statement called CONSORT (Consolidation of the Standards of Reporting Trials), which resulted from an extensive collaborative process with the aim of improving the standard of written reports of RCTs.[22] The CONSORT statement was designed to assist the reporting of RCTs with two groups and those with parallel designs. Some modifications will be required to report crossover trials and those with more than two groups.[23]

The CONSORT statement includes a checklist of 21 items and a flow diagram for use by the authors to provide journal editors and peer-reviewers with the page of the report in which each of the 21 items is addressed. The flow chart provides a detailed description of the progress of participants through the randomised trial, from the number of potentially eligible individuals for inclusion in the trial to the number of trial participants in each group who completed the trial.[23] Each of the items in the checklist and the elements of the flow chart are described in detail in Chapter 5.

Will the quality of RCTs improve?

Soon after its publication, the CONSORT statement was endorsed by major journals such as the *British Medical Journal*, *The Lancet*, the *Journal of the American Medical Association*, and the *Canadian Medical Association Journal*. These journals incorporated the CONSORT statement as part of the requirements for authors from 1 January 1997. Within six months of the publication of the statement, another 30 journals endorsed it.

Although the CONSORT statement was not evaluated before its publication, it is expected that it will lead to an improvement in the quality of reporting of RCTs, at least in the journals that have endorsed it. It is also expected that the actual quality of the trials will improve as a result of authors being aware of the requirements for submission of trial reports.

The overall effect of CONSORT and other initiatives to improve the quality of RCTs is hard to predict, taking into account that there are more than 30 000 biomedical journals and that their number is likely to continue increasing exponentially.[25] Whether there is a substantial improvement in the overall quality of future trials will depend on the extent to which researchers and editors agree that there is a need to improve their quality and are willing to make the necessary efforts to improve it.

1 Jadad AR, Moore RA, Carroll D, Jenkinson C, Reynolds JM, Gavaghan DJ, McQuay DM. Assessing the quality of reports on randomized clinical trials: Is blinding necessary? *Controlled Clin Trials* 1996;**17**:1–12.

2 Moher D, Jadad AR, Tugwell P. Assessing the quality of randomized controlled trials. *Int J Technol Assess Health Care* 1996;**12**:195–208.

3 Streiner DL, Norman GR. *Health measurement scales: a practical guide to their development and use*, 2nd edn. Oxford: Oxford University Press, 1996.

4 Schulz KF, Chalmers I, Hayes RJ, Altman DG. Empirical evidence of bias: dimensions of methodological quality associated with estimates of treatment effect in controlled clinical trials. *JAMA* 1995;**273**:408–12.

5 Chalmers TC, Celano P, Sacks HS, Smith H. Bias in treatment assignment in controlled clinical trials. *N Engl J Med* 1983;**309**:1359–61.

6 Colditz GA, Miller JN, Mosteller F. How study design affects outcomes in comparisons of therapy. I. Therapy. *Stat Med* 1989;**8**:441–54.

7 Khan KS, Daya S, Jadad AR. The importance of quality of primary studies in producing unbiased systematic reviews. *Arch Intern Med* 1996;**156**:661–6.

8 Cho MK, Bero LA. The quality of drug studies published in symposium proceedings. *Ann Intern Med* 1996;**124**:485–9.

9 Moher D, Jadad AR, Nichol G, Penman M, Tugwell P, Walsh S. Assessing the quality of randomized controlled trials: an annotated bibliography of scales and checklists. *Controlled Clin Trials* 1995;**16**:62–73.

10 Jadad AR, Cook DJ, Jones AL, Klassen TP, Tugwell P, Moher M, Moher D. The quality of randomised controlled trials included in meta-analyses and systematic reviews: how often and how is it assessed? Published as: Abstract presented at the 4th Cochrane Colloquium, Adelaide, Australia, October, 1996. *In Review at Br Med J*.

11 Jadad AR. Meta-analysis of randomised clinical trials in pain relief. DPhil thesis, University of Oxford, 1994.

12 Ohlsson A, Lacy JB. Quality assessments of randomized controlled trials: evaluation by the Chalmers versus the Jadad method. 3rd Annual Cochrane Colloquium 1995:V9–V10.

13 Egger M, Zellweger T, Antes G. Randomized trials in German-language journals. *Lancet* 1996;**347**:1047–8.

14 Bender JS, Halpern SH, Thangaroopan M, Jadad AR, Ohlsson A. Quality and retrieval of obstetrical anaesthesia randomized controlled trials. *Can J Anaesth* 1997;**44**:14–18.

15 Linde K, Clausius N, Ramirez G, Melchart D, Eitel F, Hedges LV, Jonas WB. Are the clinical effects of homeopathy placebo effects? A meta-analysis of placebo-controlled trials. *Lancet* 1997;**350**:834–43.

16 McQuay H, Carroll D, Jadad AR, Wiffen P, Moore A. Anticonvulsant drugs for management of pain: a systematic review. *BMJ* 1995;**311**:1047–52.

17 Moher D, Fortin P, Jadad AR, Juni P, Klassen T, LeLorier J, Liberati A, Linde K, Penna A. Completeness of reporting of trials published in languages other than English: implications for conduct and reporting of systematic reviews. *Lancet* 1996;**347**:363–6.

18 Egger M, Zellweger-Zahner T, Schneider M, Junker C, Lengeler C, Antes G. Language bias in randomised controlled trials published in English and German. *Lancet* 1997;**350**:326–9.

19 Moher D, Jones A, Cook DJ, Jadad AR, Moher M, Tugwell P, Klassen TP. Does the poor quality of reports of randomized trials exaggerate estimates of intervention effectiveness reported in meta-analysis? In Press. *Lancet*.

20 Berlin JA for the University of Pennsylvania Meta-analysis Blinding Study Group. Does blinding of readers affect the results of meta-analyses? *Lancet* 1997;**350**:185–6.

21 Detsky AS, Naylor CD, O'Rourke K, McGeer AJ, L'Abbe KA. Incorporating variations in the quality of individual randomized trials into meta-analysis. *J Clin Epidemiol* 1992;**45**:255–65.

22 Begg C, Cho M, Eastwood S, Horton R, Moher D, Olkin I, Pitkin R, Rennie D, Schulz KF, Simel D, Stroup D. Improving the quality of reporting of randomized controlled trials—The CONSORT Statement. *JAMA* 1996;**276**: 7–9.
23 Altman DG. Better reporting of randomised controlled trials: the CONSORT statement. *BMJ* 1996;**313**:570–1.
24 Smith R. Where is the wisdom? *BMJ* 1991;**303**:798–9.

5 Reporting and interpreting individual trials: the essentials

The extent to which you can interpret the results of a trial depends on several closely related factors, including the following:

- Your understanding of the value and limitations of RCTs as sources of information to guide decisions in health care.
- The amount and clarity of the information you find in the trial reports.
- The extent to which you are familiar with the content area addressed by the trial.
- Your understanding of the principles of data analysis and statistics.
- The time you have to read the trial report.

This book has been conceived to help you with the first two factors. This chapter will help you to identify the key elements that you should look for in a trial report to interpret its results with confidence. The other three factors—content expertise, statistical knowledge, and time—are likely to vary from reader to reader, and addressing them is obviously beyond the scope of this book.

The relationship between trial reporting and interpretation

In most cases, the only information that you will have to interpret a trial is what has been published in a journal. Unfortunately, evidence generated during the past 30 years has shown repeatedly that there is a wide gap between what a trial should report to help readers interpret their results and what is actually published.[1] Therefore, you should be prepared to find that most reports do not contain all the information that you require to make informed judgments on the internal and external validity of trials.

As described in Chapter 4, an international group of clinical epidemiologists, biostatisticians, and journal editors published, in 1996, a statement called CONSORT (Consolidation of the Standards of Reporting Trials),[1] the aim of which is to improve the standards of written reports of RCTs and to ensure that readers find in the reports all the information that they require to interpret the trial results with confidence.[2] This statement includes a checklist of 21 items and a flow diagram that authors should use to provide information on the progress of patients through a study. The original article in which the CONSORT statement was described was, however, very short and targeted authors of trial reports, not readers.[1] In this chapter, I use the CONSORT statement as a template to describe the elements that you should take into account when reading a trial report to interpret its results. I also use information from my own experience as a reader, from three series of articles produced over the past 20 years by members of the Department of Clinical Epidemiology and Biostatistics at McMaster University, and from two recent books on how to read articles.[3,4] The series includes articles on how to read clinical journals,[5-10] users' guides to the medical literature,[11,12] and a series on basic statistics for clinicians.[13-16] Table 5.1 and Fig 5.1 provide the information in CONSORT's statement. If you have not read these articles, I strongly encourage you to do so. I would also like to encourage you to get a copy of the books, which are written in friendly, easy-to-follow format.

My main challenge in writing this chapter was to keep the discussion of the issues brief and clear, focusing on the essential elements that you, the reader, need to take into account when interpreting the results of an RCT report. My aim is to help you make efficient use of the limited time you can spend reading articles. When appropriate, I expand on issues discussed in previous chapters or refer you directly to the sections of the book where certain items have been discussed in more detail. In addition, I include one or more additional sources of information where you could find detailed explanations of specific issues, particularly statistical ones, which are beyond the scope of this book.

What are the key elements of a trial report needed to interpret its results with confidence?

To interpret the results of a trial with confidence, regardless of your background, the time you have available to read a trial report,

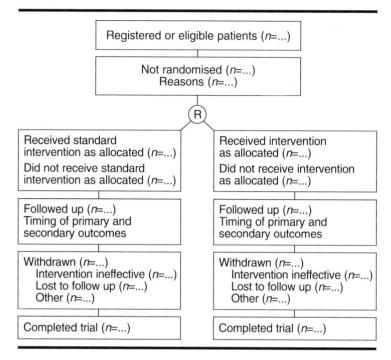

Figure 5.1 Progress through the various stages of a trial, including flow of participants, withdrawals, and timing of primary and secondary outcome measures. The "R" indicates randomisation. (From Begg et al.[1])

and the reasons why you are reading it, you will have to answer at least the following questions:

- Is the topic interesting to you?
- Are the results likely to be unbiased?
- Would you be able to use the results?
- Are the results important enough for you to remember?

In the rest of this chapter, I try to help you answer these questions in a time-efficient manner, pointing out the sections of a report in which the information you need is most likely to be found.

I am aware that you may focus on different aspects of a report: if you are a clinician trying to decide whether to use an intervention to study or treat a particular patient; if you are a researcher designing a new RCT; if you are a peer-reviewer or an editor judging whether a trial report should be published in a journal; if

Table 5.1 Consolidation of Standards for Reporting Trials—CONSORT[3,4]

Heading	Subheading	Descriptor	Was it reported?	On what page no.?
Title		Identify the study as a randomised trial[7]		
Abstract		Use a structured format[8,9]		
Introduction		State prospectively defined hypothesis, clinical objectives, and planned subgroup or co-variate analyses[10]		
Methods	Protocol	Describe		
		Planned study population, together with inclusion/exclusion criteria		
		Planned interventions and their timing		
		Primary and secondary outcome measure(s) and the minimum important difference(s), and indicate how the target sample size was projected[2,11]		
		Rationale and methods for statistical analyses, detailing main comparative analyses and whether they were completed on an intention-to-treat basis[12,13]		
		Prospectively defined stopping rules (if warranted)[14]		
	Assignment	Describe		
		Unit of randomisation (for example, individual, cluster, geographical)[15]		
		Method used to generate the allocation schedule[16]		
		Method of allocation concealment and timing of assignment[17]		
		Method to separate the generator from the executor of assignment[17,18]		
	Masking (blinding)	Describe mechanism (for example, capsules, tablets); similarity of treatment characteristics (for example, appearance, taste); allocation schedule control (location of code during trial and when broken); and evidence for successful blinding among participants, person doing intervention, outcome assessors, and data analysts[19,20]		

contd

Table 5.1 *contd*

Heading	Subheading	Descriptor	Was it reported?	On what page no.?
Results	Participant flow and follow up analysis	Provide a trial profile (see Fig 5.1) summarising participant flow, numbers, and timing of randomisation assignment, interventions, and measurements for each randomised group[3,21]		
		State estimated effect of intervention on primary and secondary outcome measures, including a point estimate and measure of precision (confidence interval)[22,23]		
		State results in absolute numbers when feasible (for example, 10/20, not 50%)		
		Present summary data and appropriate descriptive and inferential statistics in sufficient detail to permit alternative analyses and replication[24]		
		Describe prognostic variables by treatment group and any attempt to adjust for them[25]		
		Describe protocol deviations from the study as planned, together with the reasons		
Comment		State specific interpretation of study findings, including sources of bias and imprecision (internal validity) and discussion of external validity, including appropriate quantitative measures when possible		
		State general interpretation of the data in light of the totality of the available evidence		

From Begg *et al.*[1]

you are conducting a systematic review of multiple trials; if you are deciding whether to purchase a service or a new intervention; or if you are a journalist trying to decide whether to report on an article published in the latest issue of a journal. Although I do my best to provide you with enough information to answer the above questions regardless of whom you are or why you are reading a trial report, I have focused primarily on meeting the needs of busy individuals with limited experience in methodology and research.

Now, let's try to answer the questions.

Is the topic addressed by the trial interesting to you?

The answer to this question will normally depend on your background and on the degree to which the trial is likely to meet your immediate needs. For instance, a trial entitled "The use of therapeutic touch for the treatment of malignant melanoma" is likely to be interesting to you if you are an oncologist, if somebody close to you (including you, of course) has a melanoma, if you are involved in decisions about providing services for patients with melanoma, or if you are a journalist who writes about health issues.

Usually, all you need to do to establish if a report is interesting is to look at its title. If by reading the title you do not think that the article is interesting, you should either move on to another article or do something else.[5] In the rare event that you cannot find enough information in the title of a report to decide whether or not it is interesting, you are likely to find such information in the first portion of the abstract or in the introduction of the report.

After reading the title of the article, if it seems interesting, you might feel tempted to jump to the conclusions in the abstract. This may occur: because of irresistible curiosity to know the "bottom line" of the article; because your time is so limited that reading the title and parts of the abstract is all that you can do; or because you do not want to know anything else, even if you have enough time to read the whole article. I hope that, if you have read any of the previous chapters of this book (or any of the series on how to use the medical literature that I mentioned above), you understand that the information in the title and the abstract could give you a misleading message. You should use the information in an abstract just as an additional source of information to determine if the trial is interesting to you, unless you are reading journals containing only structured abstracts of high quality studies published elsewhere (see Chapter 7). You should resist the temptation to use only the information provided by the abstract of an original study to make decisions about patient care.

Are the trial results likely to be unbiased?

After spending a couple of minutes reading the title and the abstract of the trial report, if you decide that the article is still interesting, you should try to decide whether the trial is likely to be unbiased. This can be done in a simple manner by scoring the article using the three item validated scale presented in Chapter 4, by establishing whether group allocation was concealed at the time in which study participants were recruited into the study, and by looking at the sources of funding. Reports that receive a score of 2 points or less with the scale, or in which group allocation was not adequately concealed, are more likely to exaggerate the effects of the experimental intervention.[18,19] In addition, you should remember that, if a trial has been funded by industry, the report is more likely to show beneficial effects for the product of the specific company funding the trial (see Chapter 3).[20,21] As mentioned in Chapter 4, there are many other methods to assess the quality of RCTs, but none is validated, and all lack empirical evidence of their relationship to bias.[22,23]

It should take you approximately 3–5 minutes to assess the likelihood of bias in a trial report using the methods described above. With experience it could take you less than one minute, particularly if the authors have included methodological information in the title and the abstract. For example, if the title of the trial on therapeutic touch was "The use of therapeutic touch for the treatment of malignant melanoma: a randomised double-blind trial" you could not only decide whether the article is interesting, but you could also know immediately that the article describes an RCT and you could give it 2 points for being described as randomised and double-blind.

Authors of RCT reports can help you find the information you need easily, if they follow simple approaches to make the titles of their reports as informative as possible. For instance, you will have no problem finding the information you need if the authors of the report have followed an approach that has been used extensively by journals such as *ACP Journal Club* and *Evidence-Based Medicine*, two journals that have been designed to help readers access high quality information efficiently (see Chapter 7). Using this approach, efforts are made to create informative titles that tell you something not only about the topic addressed by the trial, but also about its design and results. For instance, a more informative title for the hypothetical trial on therapeutic touch for the treatment of melanoma could be "Therapeutic touch as a supplement to chemotherapy can increase survival in patients with metastatic melanoma: a randomised double-blind trial".

The abstracts of RCT reports should ideally be structured, including a systematic disclosure of the objective, research design, clinical setting, participants, interventions, main outcome measures, results, and conclusions.[24] Ideally, an abstract should contain enough information to allow you to judge how scientifically sound the trial is likely to be and how relevant its results may be to your immediate needs. If the abstract is informative enough, the information it contains should be sufficient to allow you to decide whether you should read more of the article or look at another one. As I emphasised earlier, regardless of how informative an abstract is, you should resist the temptation to use only the information provided there to make decisions about patient care.

If, based on the information in the title and abstract, you think that the trial is neither scientifically sound nor relevant to you, then you should stop reading it and, if appropriate, move to another report.

On many occasions you may think that the trial is not scientifically sound, but it is very relevant to you. In these cases, the decision as to whether to read the whole report or not should depend on the amount of additional literature available on the same topic. If you are aware of other trials addressing the same issue, then you could stop reading the report you just found. If you do not know of any other trial, however, you may want to read the whole report, very carefully, and make efforts to extract as much usable information as possible. On most occasions, such unique trials should be regarded as generators of hypotheses that you, or others, could test under more rigorous conditions.

If, based on the information in the title and abstract, you think that the trial is likely to be scientifically sound and relevant, you could decide to read the whole article from beginning to end, or to read specific components of the report in a systematic manner not only to confirm whether the trial is as scientifically sound and interesting as the title and abstract suggest, but also to determine whether you could use the results and whether the results are important enough for you to remember.

How can you determine if you would be able to use the results of a trial?

RCTs, even if perfectly designed, can tell us which treatment is better, but they cannot tell us for whom it is better. How and whether to generalise the results of an individual trial to an individual patient is one of the most complex issues in health care.[25] Perhaps the only situation in which you could apply the results of a trial to an individual is when you have done an n-of-1 trial on that individual (see Chapter 2). In the absence of an n-of-1 trial, you are left with information from a group of patients studied by others, in other patients, and in other settings. In these circumstances, you should try to determine the extent to which the research question of the trial matches your own questions, and how confident you feel based on the information available in the report about the execution and results of the trial.

Does the research question match your own questions?

As I have mentioned several times throughout the book, the research question is one of the most important components of a trial and its report. The research question is, however, frequently overlooked and underestimated by authors, peer-reviewers, and journal editors.

Under ideal circumstances, the report should include a clearly identified research question, which is formulated in simple terms and includes information on the broad characteristics of the participants (that is, male adults over 65 years of age), the condition (that is, metastatic melanoma), the setting (that is, a tertiary level cancer centre), the interventions (that is, chemotherapy alone versus chemotherapy plus therapeutic touch), and the outcomes (that is, disease-free survival, quality of life).[26] In our example, the research question could be formulated like this:

> "What is the effect of therapeutic touch as a supplement to chemotherapy compared with surgery alone on the survival rate at 5 years of adult patients with metastatic melanoma attending a tertiary level cancer centre?"

As I said before, you will not find clearly described research questions in most of the reports you read. Not finding clearly described research questions should be one of the earliest signs of concern about the report you are reading. If you do not find a clear research question, but still think that the trial could be important to you, I would encourage you to try to find as much information as possible on the individual elements of the research question in the Abstract, Introduction and Methods section of the report.

Once you have a better idea of the question or questions that the trial tried to answer, you should look for information on how the trial was executed to establish whether its results can be used by you.

Does the report include enough information on the execution of the study?

By looking for information on how the trial was executed, you will be able to judge how well it was executed and whether you could use its results. To judge the execution of a trial, you should answer the following questions.

- What was the sampling frame? How were prospective participants approached by the investigators?

    The report should provide clear information on the source of prospective participants for the trial and on the methods used to approach them. These two factors are closely related to the unit of allocation. When the unit of allocation or analysis is at the individual study participant level, the sampling frame is usually a group of patients attending a given health care institution (that is, clinics, hospitals, community centres). When groups of health professionals, special interest groups, or health care institutions themselves are the units of allocation, the sampling frame is usually a geographical area. The report should mention whether all or just a subset of all prospective participants (individuals or groups) was approached. It should also describe whether prospective participants were approached consecutively, randomly, or using any other method, and provide at least the number (and ideally the number and reasons) of prospective participants who refused to be considered for the study. If the unit of analysis of the trial is not at the individual participant level, but at a group or cluster level, the authors should provide a reason for this. In addition, if the trial used cluster randomisation (see Chapter 2), you should interpret its results carefully if the authors used standard statistical techniques, because these can lead to invalid results.[27]

Ideally, trial reports should describe prospective participants who were invited to take part in the trial but who refused to participate. This information is, however, found very rarely in trial reports.

In addition to telling you about the sources of prospective participants, the trial report should also describe how prospective participants were approached and recruited into the study. Usual methods to recruit participants include word of mouth, an invitation letter, or an advertisement in a newspaper or other media. The report should also include information on the body responsible for approving the trial from an ethical perspective (this is usually done by an institutional review board or ethics committee).

- What were the criteria used to include prospective participants or to exclude them from the study?

  The inclusion and exclusion criteria should be described in such detail that you could replicate them if you wished to do so. The description of the inclusion criteria, for instance, should provide information on the health status of the participants (that is, patients with metastatic melanoma), their previous exposure to interventions that may influence the results of the trial (that is, no previous chemotherapy, surgery, or therapeutic touch), and general demographic characteristics that could also influence the effects of the interventions (for example, age, gender, socioeconomic status, educational background, race, religious beliefs, and so on). The exclusion criteria should also be described in detail and should be justified whenever possible. The inclusion criteria are, however, often described in such detail and are so specific that a detailed description of the exclusion criteria would be unnecessary. Ideally, a report should include information on the number of prospective participants who were approached by the investigators and met the inclusion criteria but refused to participate in the study. In addition, the report should include information on prospective participants who were not included in the trial because they did not meet the inclusion criteria.

  After you identify the sources of trial participants (the sampling frame discussed in the previous question) and have a clear idea of the criteria used to select or exclude them, you should judge whether the sample studied is close enough to the population that will be affected by your decisions.

- Was the setting appropriate? Was it similar to your own setting?

  In addition to the characteristics of trial participants, you should also examine whether the setting where they were studied resembles the setting in which you have to make decisions. Therefore, the report should include information about the place where the interventions were administered (for example, both chemotherapy and therapeutic touch were conducted in a 500 bed tertiary level cancer centre affiliated with a faculty of health sciences) and where the outcomes were assessed (for example, the outcomes were assessed in the outpatient clinics of the same institution).

- What were the interventions? How and by whom were they given?

  The report should include detailed information on the characteristics of the interventions (for example, the drugs and regimens used for chemotherapy, the technique for therapeutic touch given to the patients in the experimental group and the "placebo" therapeutic touch given to patients in the control group), the profile of the individuals in charge of administering them (that is, the number, level of experience, and training of those performing all the interventions), and the regimens used to administer the interventions (usually, this refers to the number, size, and frequency of the doses of medication; in the therapeutic touch example, this could refer to the number, duration, and timing of the sessions). The report should also include information on important co-interventions (for example, the number of patients in each group who received adjuvant therapy) that could influence the outcomes of the trial.

- How were randomisation and blinding implemented?

  These two important aspects of a trial were discussed in detail in Chapter 3 and were also mentioned above in the section on assessing the likelihood of bias. In brief, the report should provide information on the method used to generate the allocation sequence, the strategies used to ensure allocation concealment, the level of blinding (masking), the methods used to blind different individuals during the trial, and whether blinding was tested. A simple way to judge whether randomisation was implemented properly is by comparing the distribution of certain characteristics of participants at the beginning of the trial (these are also called the "baseline" characteristics) across the study groups. If randomisation has been successful, there should be no statistical differences among the groups in terms of baseline characteristics thought to influence the effect of the interventions. A more detailed discussion on the presentation of data on the comparability of different study groups is found elsewhere.[28]

- What were the outcomes of interest? How were they measured?

The report should identify all outcomes that were measured during the trial, both desirable and adverse. In addition, it should specify the tools used to assess the outcomes, the time in which the outcomes were assessed, and the profile (number and background) of the people in charge of assessing them.

Once you have identified the outcomes and how they were measured, you should find out whether the authors stated which outcome was regarded as the primary one and which outcomes were regarded as secondary. The primary outcome is the main event or condition that the trial was designed to evaluate. If the primary outcome is not specified clearly or a priori (or not specified at all) and all outcomes are treated alike, there is an increased risk for the authors to highlight those with the most striking results. In addition, the more outcomes that are analysed the greater the risk of finding false positive, statistically significant results merely by chance.

- Were the results of the trial analysed properly?

This is one of the most important, complex, and yet frequently underestimated aspects of reading a trial report. Most readers typically skip sections that include statistical information, assuming that the authors, peer-reviewers, and editors have taken care of the details and have ensured that the analyses were perfect. Unfortunately, trial reports often do not provide a complete description of the statistical methods used to analyse the results and, when they do, the methods are frequently incorrectly used and applied.[29,30] Providing a detailed account of the steps and judgments that need to be made when evaluating the statistical aspects of a trial report is obviously beyond the scope of this book. Instead of overwhelming you with a myriad pieces of information that could fill a statistics book or plagiarising excellent attempts by others, I will point you to the information you should try to find in a trial report to be in a good position to judge the adequacy of the statistical analysis. With that information in hand, you could then refer to other sources that provide detailed advice, tailored to your specific needs.[4-10,31,32]

You should look for information on:

The type of data used to describe the results (for example, continuous, such as the time to death; or discrete, such as the number of deaths)

The statistical tests used (for example, t-tests, χ^2 tests, analysis of variance, and so on)

The level of statistical significance (the P values)

Efforts to estimate the sample size a priori (also known as power calculation)

The measures of the magnitude of the effects, also known as point estimates (for example, differences between the means of each group, absolute risk reduction, relative risk, odds ratio, and number needed to treat)

The confidence intervals around the point estimates (usually you will find the 95% confidence interval)

Intention-to-treat analyses (Chapter 3)

Information on subgroup analyses, ideally defined a priori (males vs females; adults vs children; White vs Afro-Americans).[33]

You should use this information to answer the following questions: If the results of the trial are positive, how likely are they to have occurred just by chance? If the results are negative, how likely is it that a true positive effect was missed?

Once you have looked for, and hopefully found, information on the methods, you should look for information on the actual results of the trial.

Does the report include enough information on the results of the trial?
Be prepared to find discrepancies between what authors planned to do, what they should have done, and what they actually report

in the Results section. In any case, you should expect the trial report to provide at least the following information:

- A profile of the flow of participants throughout the trial: the trial report should provide enough information for you to fill all the boxes in the flow chart of the CONSORT statement (see Fig 5.1). With this information, you will be able to judge the proportion of eligible participants who were actually enrolled in the trial (this will help you determine the representative nature of the study sample), the proportion of participants who received the interventions as allocated, the adequacy of follow up, the reasons why some participants were withdrawn from the study, and the number of participants who completed the trial.

- Description of the point estimates, measures of variability, and probability values for the main outcomes: often, you will find that trials report point estimates only in graphs, do not provide measures of variability (for example, confidence intervals, standard deviations, or standard errors), or do not give the actual probability values (for example, state that the results were "statistically significant" rather than the actual value of $P = 0.03$).

Once you address the previous issues and determine whether you could use the results of the trial, you should try to answer the following questions.

Is the trial important enough for you to remember and use?

This is another complex question. It may, however, be simply answered by saying that the importance of a trial and its results are in the eye of the beholder. Your decision in each case is likely to depend on: the interaction between the methodological characteristics and content of the trial itself; your own beliefs, values and preferences; and the circumstances in which you are reading the article. In all cases, however, your decision will be influenced by each of the trial characteristics discussed so far, and additional factors such as your interpretation of the magnitude of the effects of the interventions, both favourable and undesirable, found in the study.

75

Should you base your decisions on the results of a single trial?

The answer, in most cases, is likely to be no. The main reason is that, despite how interesting, relevant, unbiased, and well reported an individual trial may be, such a trial is likely to be just one among many other studies that address the same question, and which may contradict or corroborate the findings of the trial. It is, therefore, important to set the results of individual trials in the context of other relevant studies.

In the next chapter, I introduce you to different ways in which the information from a single trial can be integrated with information from other trials.

1 Begg C, Cho M, Eastwood S, Horton R, Moher D, Olkin I, Pitkin R, Rennie D, Schulz KF, Simel D, Stroup D. Improving the quality of reporting of randomized controlled trials—The CONSORT Statement. *JAMA* 1996;**276**: 7–9.
2 Altman DG. Better reporting of randomised controlled trials: the CONSORT statement. *BMJ* 1996;**313**:570–1.
3 Crombie IK. *The pocket guide to critical appraisal.* London: BMJ Publishing Group, 1996.
4 Greenhalgh T. *How to read a paper: The basics of evidence based medicine.* London: BMJ Publishing Group, 1996.
5 Department of Clinical Epidemiology and Biostatistics, McMaster University. How to read clinical journals: I. Why to read them and how to start reading them critically. *Can Med Assoc J* 1981;**124**:555–8.
6 Department of Clinical Epidemiology and Biostatistics, McMaster University. How to read clinical journals: II. To learn about a diagnostic test. *Can Med Assoc J* 1981;**124**:703–10.
7 Department of Clinical Epidemiology and Biostatistics, McMaster University. How to read clinical journals: III. To learn about the clinical course and prognosis of disease. *Can Med Assoc J* 1981;**124**:869–79.
8 Department of Clinical Epidemiology and Biostatistics, McMaster University. How to read clinical journals: IV. To determine the etiology or causation of disease. *Can Med Assoc J* 1981;**124**:985–90.
9 Department of Clinical Epidemiology and Biostatistics, McMaster University. How to read clinical journals: V. To distinguish useful from useless or even harmful therapy. *Can Med Assoc J* 1981;**124**:1156–62.
10 Department of Clinical Epidemiology and Biostatistics, McMaster University. How to read clinical journals: VI. To learn about the quality of clinical care. *Can Med Assoc J* 1984;**130**:377–81.
11 Guyatt GH, Sackett DL, Cook DJ for the Evidence-Based Medicine Working Group. Users' guides to the medical literature. II. How to use an article about therapy or prevention. A. Are the results of the study valid? *JAMA* 1993;**270**: 2598–601.
12 Guyatt GH, Sackett DL, Cook DJ for the Evidence-Based Medicine Working Group. Users' guides to the medical literature. II. How to use an article about

therapy or prevention. B. What were the results and will they help me in caring for my patients? *JAMA* 1994;**271**:59–63.

13 Guyatt G, Jaeschke R, Heddle N, Cook D, Shannon H, Walter S. Basic statistics for clinicians: 1. Hypothesis testing. *Can Med Assoc J* 1995;**152**:27–32.

14 Guyatt G, Jaeschke R, Heddle N, Cook D, Shannon H, Walter S. Basic statistics for clinicians: 2. Interpreting study results: confidence intervals. *Can Med Assoc J* 1995;**152**:169–73.

15 Guyatt G, Walter S, Shannon H, Cook D, Jaeschke R, Heddle N. Basic statistics for clinicians: 4. Correlation and regression. *Can Med Assoc J* 1995;**152**:497–504.

16 Jaeschke R, Guyatt G, Shannon H, Walter S, Cook D, Heddle N. Basic statistics for clinicians: 3. Assessing the effects of treatment: measures of association. *Can Med Assoc J* 1995;**152**:351–7.

17 Jadad AR, Moore RA, Carroll D, Jenkinson C, Reynolds JM, Gavaghan DJ, McQuay DM. Assessing the quality of reports on randomized clinical trials: Is blinding necessary? *Controlled Clin Trials* 1996;**17**:1–12.

18 Moher D, Jones A, Cook DJ, Jadad AR, Moher M, Tugwell P, Klassen TP. Does the poor quality of reports of randomized trials exaggerate estimates of intervention effectiveness reported in meta-analysis? *In press, Lancet.*

19 Schulz KF, Chalmers I, Hayes RJ, Altman DG. Empirical evidence of bias: dimensions of methodological quality associated with estimates of treatment effect in controlled clinical trials. *JAMA* 1995;**273**:408–12.

20 Cho MK, Bero LA. The quality of drug studies published in symposium proceedings. *Ann Intern Med* 1996;**124**:485–9.

21 Gotszche PC. Methodology and overt and hidden bias in reports of 196 double-blind trials of nonsteroidal antiinflammatory drugs in rheumatoid arthritis. *Controlled Clin Trials* 1989;**10**:31–56.

22 Moher D, Jadad AR, Nichol G, Penman M, Tugwell P, Walsh S. Assessing the quality of randomized controlled trials: an annotated bibliography of scales and checklists. *Controlled Clin Trials* 1995;**16**:62–73.

23 Jadad AR, Cook DJ, Jones AL, Klassen TP, Tugwell P, Moher M, Moher D. The quality of randomised controlled trials included in meta-analyses and systematic reviews: how often and how is it assessed? Published as: Abstract presented at the 4th Cochrane Colloquium, Adelaide, Australia, October 1996. *In Review at Br Med J.*

24 Haynes RB, Mulrow CD, Huth EJ, Altman DG, Gardner MJ. More informative abstracts revisited. *Ann Intern Med* 1990;**113**:69–76.

25 Bailey KR. Generalizing the results of randomized clinical trials. *Controlled Clin Trials* 1994;**15**:15–23.

26 Richardson W, Wilson M, Nishikawa J, Hayward RSA. The well-built clinical question: a key to evidence-based decisions. *ACP J Club* 1995;**123**:12–13.

27 Donner A, Brown KS, Brasher P. A methodological review of non-therapeutic intervention trials employing cluster randomization, 1979–1989. *Int J Epidemiol* 1990;**19**:795–800.

28 Altman DG. Comparability of randomized groups. *Statistician* 1985;**34**:125–36.

29 Evans M, Pollock AV. Trials on trial: a review of trials of antibiotic prophylaxis. *Arch Surg* 1984;**119**:109–13.

30 Gardner MJ, Bond J. An exploratory study of statistical assessment of papers published in the *British Medical Journal*. *JAMA* 1990;**263**:1355–7.

31 Altman DG. *Practical statistics for medical research*. London: Chapman & Hall, 1991.

32 Streiner DL, Norman GR. *PDQ epidemiology*, 2nd edn. St Louis: CV Mosby, 1996.

33 Oxman AD, Guyatt GH. A consumer's guide to subgroup analysis. *Ann Intern Med* 1992;**116**:78–84.

6 From individual trials to groups of trials: reviews, meta-analyses, and guidelines

Often you will find more than one trial that addresses your question or a very similar research question. As these trials are conducted in different groups of people, in different settings, and use the interventions differently, it is unlikely that they will provide identical results. Sometimes, different trials on the same topic have totally opposite results. The corollary is that it may be risky for you and for your patients to make decisions based on the information from a single trial. If you want to make decisions based on the best available knowledge, I am sure that you would like to consider as many relevant trials as possible. You will also want to take into account other types of information (see Chapter 7). Identifying and synthesising the information from all relevant trials to guide a particular decision are not, however, easy tasks. In this chapter, I introduce you to the identification of trials and the role of reviews of multiple trials to guide health care decisions. As in previous chapters, most of the issues that I discuss deserve a chapter and have been addressed more extensively elsewhere. My intention here, as in the rest of the book, is to highlight the most relevant information, directing you to more comprehensive sources that you could consult at your own convenience. Let's start.

What are the main impediments to identifying all relevant trials on a given topic?

The main problem derives from the speed with which the literature is growing. It has been estimated, for example, that over 2 million articles and more than 17 000 biomedical books are published annually.[1,2] It is difficult to estimate the total number of trials that have been completed to date, but it is thought to be in the hundreds of thousands.[3] In some areas, the time it takes for the number of published trials to double is less than 10 years.[4]

This information "explosion" is compounded by the fact that there is not a single source of information that could provide easy and reliable access to all randomised controlled trials (RCTs) on a given topic. All existing databases are incomplete (one of the main problems being the poor access to unpublished trials) and use coding systems that cannot cope with the diversity of topics in health care.

What is the best source of RCTs?

Perhaps the most advanced and comprehensive source of RCTs in health care is the Cochrane Controlled Trials Database, which contains citations for more than 150 000 controlled trials identified through the collective effort of members of the Cochrane Collaboration (see below) to improve the identification of primary studies. This has been achieved not only through the development of high yield strategies to search bibliographic databases, but also through extensive hand searching of journals to identify studies that cannot be identified efficiently by electronic searches or that are not indexed in bibliographic databases. The complete database is available on CD-ROM and is updated four times a year. More information on this database and other products of the Cochrane Collaboration can be obtained from the Internet at: http://hiru.mcmaster.ca/cochrane.

Other sources of information that you could use to identify citations of RCTs are traditional bibliographic databases such as MEDLINE or EMBASE. You can now search MEDLINE, free of charge, on the Internet. There are many providers of access to MEDLINE, but you may want to access it directly through the US National Library of Medicine at http://ncbi.nlm.nih.gov/PubMed. At this site, you could access using search strategies specifically designed to optimise the yield of clinically useful studies. To access these strategies, go to http://ncbi.nlm.nih.gov/PubMed/clinical.html. You can also access MEDLINE through other vendors that provide more comprehensive and expensive services, including access to full text articles.[5]

Even if you identify citations for all the studies you require to inform a particular decision, an additional problem is the time required to obtain hard copies of the articles and to read

79

them. Sometimes, key articles are published in languages that you may not understand. You would have to ignore them or invest resources to have them translated. You will have to face all these problems if you decide to identify the trials on your own. On the other hand, you may choose to explore other options that could facilitate your efforts to identify and synthesise multiple trials.

Are there ways to make it easier to find and use multiple RCTs?

Fortunately, there are several options that can give you access to information from many trials with less effort and hassle. One of these options is to read a summary prepared by others, relying on those who have already spent time, money, and energy to summarise information from multiple trials on the topic. Alternatively, you could join a group of people with common interests and review a particular topic or group of topics with them, sharing the workload and resources. In the following sections, I concentrate on review articles in general, highlighting the different types of reviews and their strengths and weaknesses.

What are the different types of reviews?

As a result of the rapid expansion of the literature and the progressive compression of our time and resources, review articles are becoming increasingly attractive tools to guide health care decisions. As with any other tools, however, reviews can be well built or defective, and can be well used or abused.

In theory, there are two major types of reviews: narrative and systematic. In practice, most reviews share elements of these two major types. These reviews may consider only RCTs, or RCTs and other study designs. In this chapter, I discuss some general principles of reviews, but focus on reviews of RCTs. In Chapter 7, I introduce you to the relationship between RCTs and other study designs, as well as other sources of information.

What is a narrative review?

A narrative review is the typical review article that you find in most journals. These reviews are produced by individuals who are often considered to be experts in a given field, using idiosyncratic, often informal and subjective, methods to collect and interpret information. They appeal to reviewers because they are relatively easy and quick to produce. They are also attractive to readers because they distil the views of an authority in a field in a short piece, saving the readers time and effort. The main problem with these reviews, however, is that the reader must take them at face value, because they are impossible to replicate. This could be a real problem in an era of information overload in which we make increasingly complex decisions and need to be increasingly accountable. In fact, it has been shown recently that narrative reviews are not only incomplete, [6] but that they can delay the identification of effective or harmful interventions by 10–15 years when compared with more systematic approaches to reviewing the literature.[7,8]

What is a systematic review?

A systematic review, in its ideal form, is a review that includes an explicit and detailed description of how it was conducted so that any interested reader would be able to replicate it. The ideal systematic review should incorporate strategies to minimise bias and to maximise precision. In its purest form, the report of a systematic review should include a clear research question, criteria for inclusion or exclusion of primary studies, the process used to identify primary studies, the methods used to assess the methodological quality of the selected studies, and the methods used to extract and summarise the results of primary trials on which the conclusions are based.[9] Entire series of articles devoted to systematic reviews have been published recently in major peer-reviewed journals (worth mentioning are series published by the *British Medical Journal* in 1994 and by the *Annals of Internal Medicine* in 1997).

Systematic reviews clearly overcome the major limitations of narrative reviews. Their main disadvantage is that they require more time and resources to prepare than do their narrative counterparts.

What is meta-analysis?

Meta-analysis is a name that is given to any review article in which the results of several independent studies are combined statistically to produce a single estimate of the effect of a particular intervention or health care situation. In other words, the results

81

of independent studies are lumped together to produce a number or a graph (usually with confidence intervals) that summarises the effect of the intervention. Other names given to meta-analysis include overview, quantitative overview, pooling, pooled analysis, integrative research review, research integration, research consolidation, data synthesis, quantitative synthesis, and combining studies.[10]

The main purpose of meta-analysis is to increase the precision of the conclusions of a review. This increased precision could do the following:

- Make comparisons of interventions more objective and accurate.
- Help resolve controversies arising from studies with conflicting results.
- Enable clinicians and patients to make better decisions.
- Guide clinical research by generating new hypotheses.
- Identify areas in which insufficient research has been performed or in which additional research may not be necessary.

Meta-analyses also have limitations. Some of these limitations result from the limitations of the individual RCTs that they combine, because the trials could have insufficient sample sizes, biased designs, be reported incompletely, or try to answer irrelevant questions. Other limitations arise from the way in which meta-analyses are designed and conducted. Meta-analyses, for example, could be prone to bias of many types and from many sources. A catalogue of the biases that can affect meta-analyses was compiled recently and is presented elsewhere,[11] and empirical evidence is emerging to support their existence and importance.[12–14] Another limitation of meta-analyses is that they usually require the use of statistical techniques that are still poorly understood by reviewers and readers. A useful description of procedures used in meta-analyses was published recently and I would encourage you to read it.[15] The BMJ also published a series of articles on meta-analysis in 1997 and 1998.

Are systematic reviews and meta-analysis the same thing?

Even though most people use the terms interchangeably, systematic reviews and meta-analyses are not synonyms. Let's elaborate on this a little.

How can a systematic review not be a meta-analysis?

A review may incorporate state-of-the-art strategies to minimise bias and to maximise precision, but, at the end, the reviewer may decide that the results of the RCTs included should not be combined. Data combination may be inappropriate for many reasons. For example, the trials may be too different in terms of their eligibility criteria, interventions, outcome time-points, the volume of data available, or methodological quality. Assessing how much heterogeneity exists among trials included in a review and assessing whether they should be combined make up one of the crucial steps in a systematic review. If, after evaluating the characteristics of the included trials, the reviewer decides that the trials can be combined, the systematic review includes meta-analysis and could also be called a systematic *quantitative* review. If a decision is made against combining the trials, the review is still systematic and should perhaps be called a systematic *qualitative* review. These two terms are important for two reasons: first, they define the distinction between meta-analyses that do and do not result from a systematic and scientific review process; and, second, they highlight the fact that not all systematic processes for reviewing a particular body of scientific evidence should necessarily lead to the statistical combination of data across studies.

Is it possible to use meta-analysis in a review that is not systematic?

The minimum requirement to produce a meta-analysis is the availability of data from two or more studies, irrespective of whether they are being reviewed narratively or systematically. For instance, a reviewer may decide to combine data from two studies that he found on top of his desk on the morning he was to submit the review for publication. In this case, the resulting review could be called a meta-analysis, but it would be far from a systematic review.

Multiple studies during the past decade have shown consistently that most meta-analyses published in peer-reviewed journals lack several of the components of a rigorous systematic review.[13,16-18] In response to this evidence, multiple efforts are being made to improve the methodological quality of meta-analyses. Perhaps the most important effort is that of an initiative known as QUOROM (Quality of Reporting Meta-analyses), which is similar to the

Oxman and Guyatt's index of the scientific quality of research overviews

The purpose of this index is to evaluate the scientific quality (i.e. adherence to scientific principles) of research overviews (review articles) published in the medical literature. It is not intended to measure literary quality, importance, relevance, originality, or other attributes of overviews.

The index is for assessing overviews of primary ('original') research on pragmatic questions regarding causation, diagnosis, prognosis, therapy or prevention. A research overview is a survey of research. The same principles that apply to epidemiologic survey apply to overviews: a question must be clearly specified, a target population identified and accessed, appropriate information obtained from that population in an unbiased fashion, and conclusions derived, sometimes with the help of formal statistical analysis, as is done in 'meta-analyses'. The fundamental difference between overviews and epidemiologic surveys is the unit of analysis, not the scientific issues that the questions in this index address.

Since most published overviews do not include a methods section it is difficult to answer some of the questions in the index. Base your answers, as much as possible, on the information provided in the overview. If the methods that were used are reported incompletely relative to a specific item, score that item as 'partially'. Similarly, if there is no information provided regarding what was done relative to a particular question, score it as 'can't tell', unless there is information in the overview to suggest either that the criterion was or was not met.

1. Were the search methods used to find evidence (original research) on the primary question(s) stated?
   ❑ yes   ❑ partially   ❑ no

Yes is given to meta-analysis reporting categories of sources, including years [e.g. databases-medline] used, and whether these categories were explained. Partial points are given for the category of sources and how many of the categories [e.g. electronic, hand, register] are named.

2. Was the search for evidence reasonably comprehensive?
   ❑ yes   ❑ can't tell   ❑ no

Yes is given if at least three categories, one of which must be electronic with key words stated, and any two others [e.g. hand, register] are reported. Key words and/or MESH terms must be stated.

3. Were the criteria used for deciding which studies to include in the overview reported?
   ❑ yes   ❑ partially   ❑ no

This item was thought to be reasonably explicit.

4. Was bias in the selection of studies avoided?
   ❑ yes   ❑ can't tell   ❑ no

Yes is given if at least two reviewers independently assess for inclusion. A consensus must be reached.

5. Were the criteria used for assessing the validity of the included studies reported?
   ❏ yes   ❏ partially   ❏ no

It was felt that the issues relating to publication bias should not be included in the assessment of this. Yes is given to those meta-analysis reporting 'a priori' methods of validity assessment.

6. Was the validity of all studies referred to in the text assessed using appropriate criteria (either in selecting studies for inclusion or in analyzing the studies that are cited)?
   ❏ yes   ❏ can't tell   ❏ no

This item relates to validity assessment. Yes is given if there is a description of any criteria [either internal or external] used.

7. Were the methods used to combine the findings of the relevant studies (to reach a conclusion) reported?
   ❏ yes   ❏ partially   ❏ no

This item was thought to be reasonably explicit.

8. Were the findings of the relevant studies combined appropriately relative to the primary question the overview addresses?
   ❏ yes   ❏ can't tell   ❏ no

For question 8, if no attempt was made to combine findings, and no statement is made regarding the inappropriateness of combining findings, check 'no'. If a summary (general) estimate is given anywhere in the abstract, the discussion or the summary section of the paper, and it is not reported how the estimate was derived, mark 'no' even if there is a statement regarding the limitations of combining the findings of the studies reviewed. If in doubt mark 'can't tell'.

9. Were the conclusions made by the author(s) supported by the data and/or analysis reported in the overview?
   ❏ yes   ❏ partially   ❏ no

For an overview to be scored as 'yes' on question 9, data (not just citations) must be reported that supports the main conclusions regarding the primary question(s) that the overview addresses.

10. How would you rate the scientific quality of the overview?

extensive flaws		major flaws		minor flaws		minimal flaws
❏	❏	❏	❏	❏	❏	❏
1	2	3	4	5	6	7

The score for question 10, the overall scientific quality, should be based on your answers to the first nine questions. The following guidelines can be used to assist with deriving a summary score. If the 'can't tell' option is used one or more times on the preceding questions, a review is likely to have minor flaws at best and it is difficult to rule out major flaws (i.e. a score of 4 or lower). If the 'no' option is used on question 2, 4, 6 or 8, the review is likely to have major flaws (i.e. a score of 3 or less, depending on the number and degree of the flaws).

Figure 6.1   Oxman and Guyatt's index of the scientific quality of research overviews.[19] (From Jadad and McQuay.[13])

CONSORT efforts to improve the quality of randomised trials. For more information on QUOROM, you can contact the coordinating office at the University of Ottawa (David Moher, Children's Hospital of Eastern Ontario Research Institute, 401 Smyth Road, Ottawa, Ontario, K1H 8L1, Canada).

Needless to say, inappropriate meta-analyses may result in more harm than good. Reviewers should understand that a systematic qualitative review of the literature, in its own right, is a more effective way to summarise the evidence than an inappropriate or misleading meta-analysis.

How can you evaluate the quality of a review?

The assessment of the quality of reviews, whether narrative or systematic, has the same challenges as the assessment of the quality of individual trials (see Chapter 4). There are several published instruments for assessing the quality of reviews, but only one has been extensively validated,[19] and published elsewhere.[13] This instrument, with slightly modified instructions, is shown in Fig 6.1. Modifications in the instructions were made during the course of several empirical methodological studies to maximise interrater agreement. Another version of the instrument, in this case with major modifications, is included as part of the "Users' guides to the medical literature".[20]

Do reviews on the same topic always agree?

As the number of published systematic reviews increases, you will often find more than one systematic review addressing the same or a very similar therapeutic question. Despite the promise for systematic reviews to resolve conflicting results generated by primary studies, conflicts among reviews are now emerging. These conflicts produce difficulties for decision makers who rely on these reviews to help them make choices among alternative health interventions where experts and individual trials disagree. In a recent article, I proposed a tool in the form of a decision algorithm that I developed with two of my colleagues at McMaster, which could help in the interpretation of discordant reviews (Fig 6.2).[21]

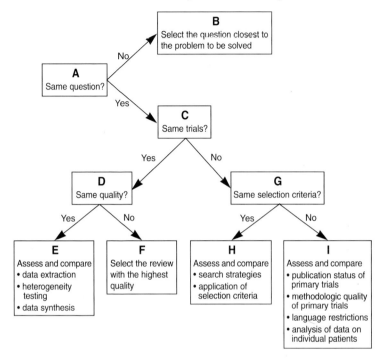

Figure 6.2 A decision algorithm for interpreting discordant reviews (assuming that the reviews have few and minimal flaws). (From Jadad et al.[21])

Can rigorous reviews eliminate the need for further trials?

This is one of the most controversial and complex issues in health care research today. The controversy goes on throughout a continuum. At one end are those who insist that if a rigorous meta-analysis shows evidence of effectiveness or harm for an intervention, it would be unethical to conduct another study.[7] At the other end are those who regard meta-analysis, particularly of small trials, as untrustworthy and advocate for rigorous mega-trials to determine the effectiveness or harm of health care interventions.[22] This controversy has been fuelled recently by the publication of several studies showing frequent discrepancies in the results of meta-analyses of small trials and large randomised controlled trials.[14,23-25] Possible reasons for the discordance between meta-analyses and large trials include major differences in the protocols and research questions, publication bias, and the inclusion of patient populations with different levels of risk in small and large trials.[23]

What is the role of the Cochrane Collaboration in all this?

The Cochrane Collaboration is an international organisation that aims to help people make informed decisions about health, by preparing, maintaining, and ensuring the accessibility of rigorous, systematic, and up to date reviews (and, where possible, meta-analyses) of the benefits and risks of health care interventions.[26–29] It was founded at a meeting of about 80 people from several countries who gathered in Oxford, England, in the fall of 1993.[28] The Collaboration is named after a physician–epidemiologist, Archie Cochrane, who more than 15 years ago criticised the medical profession for not having organised "a critical summary, by specialty or subspecialty, adapted periodically, of all relevant randomised controlled trials" to guide their clinical decisions.[30]

Since its creation, the Cochrane Collaboration has undergone an unprecedented growth. The Collaboration holds such promise to facilitate health care decision making that it has been described as "an enterprise that rivals the Human Genome Project in its potential implications for modern medicine".[31] Nevertheless, this rapidly developing organisation is also experiencing "growing pains" and facing important challenges.[29] The structure of the Collaboration, and its recent achievements and challenges, are described elsewhere.[32]

The main product of the Cochrane Collaboration is the Cochrane Library. As mentioned above, this is a regularly updated electronic library designed to give decision makers the evidence they need to make informed health care decisions, with special emphasis on data from RCTs. Launched in April 1995 as the Cochrane Database of Systematic Reviews (CDSR), it was renamed to reflect the inclusion of additional, important, related databases, making it perhaps the most comprehensive source of evidence for all those interested in evidence based health care (see Chapter 7). The Cochrane Library is issued quarterly and contains general information on the Cochrane Collaboration, a handbook on how to conduct systematic reviews, and the following four databases.[32]

The Cochrane Database of Systematic Reviews (CDSR)   This is a rapidly growing collection of regularly updated systematic reviews of the effects of health care prepared by members of Collaborative Review Groups. It also includes protocols of reviews in progress.

The Database of Abstracts of Reviews of Effectiveness (DARE)   This is a database of structured abstracts of thousands of systematic reviews from around the world, all of which have been completed outside of the Cochrane Collaboration. These reviews have been approved by reviewers at the National Health Service Centre for Reviews and Dissemination at the University of York, England. DARE also includes brief records of reviews that may be useful for background information, abstracts of reports of health technology agencies world wide, and abstracts of reviews in the journals *ACP Journal Club* and *Evidence-Based Medicine* (see Chapter 7).

The Cochrane Controlled Trials Register   See above for information.

The Cochrane Review Methodology Database (CRMD)   This is a database that contains hundreds of citations of articles on the science of research synthesis and on practical aspects of preparing systematic reviews.

The Cochrane Library is available on CD-ROM for Windows and Macintosh and should be regarded as an evolving product. More details on the Cochrane Library and on distributors can be found on the Internet: http://hiru.mcmaster.ca/cochrane.

Should systematic reviews include only RCTs?

Even though most systematic reviews in health care focus on therapy and RCTs, the same approach could and should be used to summarise information produced in any other area of health care and by any other type of study design. It is still unclear, however, whether and how to use meta-analysis to complement systematic reviews in areas other than therapy (that is, diagnostics, screening, natural history, health economics) and for studies other than RCTs.

What is the difference between systematic reviews and clinical practice guidelines?

Clinical practice guidelines have been defined as "systematically developed statements to assist practitioner and patient decisions about appropriate health care for specific clinical circumstances".[33] These statements are usually presented as "recommendations" for clinical practice and policy. Clinical practice guidelines represent a step beyond systematic reviews when their recommendations integrate research evidence from systematic reviews with the values and preferences of the developers of the guidelines and the context in which the guidelines will be applied. Systematic reviews should not include recommendations for practice or policy, but should be limited to providing a summary of the data available in the studies included and perhaps only suggestions for practice and research. Instead, they should be used as a component of clinical practice guidelines, providing the "evidence base" from which recommendations are derived. Despite this, do not be surprised if you find systematic reviews with very strong recommendations for clinical practice and policy.

Apart from an explicit process for deriving guidelines from the evidence, guidelines should consider all important management options. Guidelines on attention deficit/hyperactivity disorder, for example, should not simply look at the role of stimulants, given that there are other treatment options, including other pharmacological (for example, antidepressants) and non-pharmacological (for example, dietary, behavioural, or cognitive) therapies. Guidelines should also provide information on the strength of the evidence in support of a recommendation and the extent of the potential impact on clinical practice and policy if the recommendation is implemented.[34]

Developing guidelines necessarily involves relatively small numbers of people with a limited range of views and skills. This is why it is important that the recommendations from such groups be evaluated and modulated by external review and comment from others who are interested in the problems addressed by the guidelines (for example, a wide range of practitioners, managers, policy makers, and patients or their representatives) and tested in the field in which they are to be implemented.

Many practitioners distrust practice guidelines, and it is true that some guidelines should be distrusted. As with any other tool, including RCTs and systematic reviews, guidelines can be misused, especially when they are not based on a rigorous and objective analysis of current best evidence or when they are used in settings very different from the one in which they were developed. An increasing number of guidelines, however, provide practical recommendations based on sound evidence. Some, quite appropriately, even incorporate feedback from practitioners, and provide separate clinical and policy recommendations.[35] These sound evidence based guidelines can help practitioners to improve the care that they offer their patients.

1 Mulrow CD. Rationale for systematic reviews. In: Chalmers I, Altman DG, eds. *Systematic reviews*. London: BMJ Publishing Group, 1995;1–8.
2 Lowe HJ, Barnett O. Understanding and using the medical subject subheadings (MeSH) vocabulary to perform literature searches. *JAMA* 1994;**271**:1103–8.
3 Jadad AR, Rennie D. The randomized controlled trial gets a middle-aged checkup. *JAMA* 1998;**279**:319–20.
4 Jadad AR, Carroll D, Moore RA, McQuay HJ. Developing a database of published reports of randomised clinical trials in pain research. *Pain* 1996;**66**: 239–46.
5 Haynes RB, Jadad AR, Hunt DL. What's up in medical informatics? *Can Med Assoc J* 1997;**157**:1718–19.
6 Hillier TLB, Jadad AR. The development of a database on the measurement of pain. *Supportive Care in Cancer* 1996;**3**:246.
7 Lau J, Antman EM, Jimenez-Silva J, Kupelnick B, Mosteller F, Chalmers TC. Cumulative meta-analysis of therapeutic trials for myocardial infarction. *N Engl J Med* 1992;**327**:248–54.
8 Antman EM, Lau J, Kupelnick B, Mosteller F, Chalmers TC. A comparison of results of meta-analyses of randomized control trials and recommendations of clinical experts. *JAMA* 1992;**268**:240–8.
9 Oxman AD, Guyatt GH. Guidelines for reading literature reviews. *Can Med Assoc J* 1988;**138**:697–703.
10 Jenicek M. Meta-analysis in medicine: where we are and where we want to go. *J Clin Epidemiol* 1989;**42**:35–44.
11 Felson DT. Bias in meta-analytic research. *J Clin Epidemiol* 1992;**45**:885–92.
12 Simes RJ. Confronting publication bias: a cohort design for meta-analysis. *Statist Med* 1987;**6**:11–29.
13 Jadad AR, McQuay HJ. Meta-analysis to evaluate analgesic interventions: a systematic qualitative review of their methodology. *J Clin Epidemiol* 1996;**49**: 235–43.
14 Egger M, Smith GD, Schneider M, Minder C. Bias in meta-analysis detected by a simple, graphical test. *BMJ* 1997;**315**:629–34.
15 Lau J, Ioannidis JPA, Schmid CH. Quantitative synthesis in systematic reviews. *Ann Inter Med* 1997;**127**:820–6.
16 Jadad AR, Cook DJ, Jones A, Klassen TP, Tugwell P, Moher M, Moher D. Methodology and reports of systematic reviews and meta-analyses: a comparison of Cochrane reviews with articles published in paper-based journals. *JAMA* 1998;**280**.
17 Assendelft WJJ, Koes BW, Knipschild PG, Bouter LM. The relationship between methodological quality and conclusions in reviews of spinal manipulation. *JAMA* 1995;**274**:1942–8.

18 Sacks HS, Berrier J, Reitman D, Pagano D, Chalmers T. Meta-analyses of randomized control trials: An update of the quality and methodology. In: Bailar JC III, Mosteller F, eds. *Medical uses of statistics*. Boston, MA: New England Medical Journal Publications, 1992;427–42.

19 Oxman AD, Guyatt GH. Validation of an index of the quality of review articles. *J Clin Epidemiol* 1991;**44**:1271–8.

20 Oxman AD, Cook DJ, Guyatt GH for the Evidence-Based Medicine Working Group. Users' guides to the medical literature. VI. How to use an overview. *JAMA* 1994;**272**:1367–71.

21 Jadad AR, Cook D, Browman GP. When arbitrators disagree: a guide to interpreting discordant systematic reviews of health care interventions. *Can Med Assoc J* 1997;**156**:1411–16.

22 Bailar JC III. The promise and problems of meta-analysis. *N Engl J Med* 1997; **337**:559–60.

23 Cappelleri JC, Ioannidis JPA, Schmid CH, de Ferranti SD, Aubert M, Chalmers TC, Lau J. Large trials vs meta-analysis of smaller trials: How do their results compare? *JAMA* 1996;**276**:1332–8.

24 LeLorier J, Gregoire, G, Benhaddad A, Lapierre J, Derderian F. Discrepancies between meta-analyses and subsequent large randomized, controlled trials. *N Engl J Med* 1997;**337**:536–42.

25 Villar J, Carroli G, Pelizan JM. Predictive ability of meta-analyses of randomised controlled trials. *Lancet* 1995;**345**:772–6.

26 Godlee F. The Cochrane Collaboration. *Br Med J* 1994;**309**:969–70.

27 Sackett DL. The Cochrane Collaboration. *ACP Journal Club* 1994;May/June: A-11.

28 Bero L, Rennie D. The Cochrane Collaboration: preparing, maintaining, and disseminating systematic reviews of the effects of health care. *JAMA* 1995;**274**: 1935–8.

29 Huston P. Cochrane Collaboration helping unravel tangled web woven by international research. *Can Med Assoc J* 1996;**154**:1389–92.

30 Cochrane AL. *1931–1971: a critical review, with particular reference to the medical profession*. London: Office of Health Economics, 1979.

31 Naylor CD. Grey zones of clinical practice: some limits to evidence-based medicine. *Lancet* 1995;**345**:840–2.

32 Jadad AR, Haynes RB. The Cochrane Collaboration—Advances and challenges in improving evidence-based decision making. *Medical Decision Making* 1998; **18**:2–9.

33 Field MJ, Lohr KN (eds). *Clinical practice guidelines: Directions for a new program. Institute of Medicine*. Washington, DC: National Academy Press, 1990.

34 Guyatt GH, Sackett DL, Sinclair JC, Hayward R, Cook DJ, Cook RJ for the Evidence-based Medicine Working Group. Users' guides to the medical literature. IX. A method for grading health care recommendations. *JAMA* 1995;**274**:1800–4.

35 Browman GP, Levine MN, Mohide EA, Hayward RSA, Pritchard KI, Gafni A, Laupacis A. The practice guidelines development cycle: a conceptual tool for practice guidelines development and implementation. *J Clin Oncol* 1995;**13**: 502–12.

7 From trials to decisions: the basis of evidence based health care

Health care decisions are usually the result of the interaction of the information available to the decision makers, their values and preferences, and the circumstances or context in which the decisions are made.[1] Randomised controlled trials (RCTs), even if assembled into a perfect systematic review, are just one of the many different types of information that can inform decisions. In this chapter, I describe the different types of information that can influence the role of RCTs in decision making, and how such information can be processed, modulated, and integrated into decisions, according to different values, preferences, and circumstances.

What types of information can be used to make health care decisions?

Decisions can be influenced by formal research studies or by anecdotal information. By anecdotal information I mean any type of information informally gained, from either personal or clinical experiences, one's own or that of others, without the use of formal research methodology.[2]

If you want to understand the role of RCTs in decision making, it is crucial that you recognise that RCTs are just one of many different types of research studies, and that research studies are just one type of information. You should also realise that the interaction between different types of information in health care decision making is perhaps as complex and poorly understood as the interaction of information, values, preferences, and circumstances. The obvious first step to exploring this interaction is a basic understanding of the different types of information that you can use to make decisions. Let's start with formal research.

What are the different types of research studies?

Research studies can be either quantitative or qualitative.

What is a quantitative study?

A quantitative study is one that presents its results using numbers. Studies are called experimental if investigators influence the way in which the interventions are administered. RCTs are obviously the most important type of experimental study. This group also includes controlled clinical trials in which participants are allocated to the study groups using methods other than randomisation (see Chapter 1).

When the investigators do not influence the course of the events, the studies are called observational. These studies can be controlled or non-controlled and, depending on how the data are gathered in time, they can be prospective, retrospective, or cross sectional. The controlled observational studies can be classified further into those with contemporaneous controls (studies in which data from the different groups are obtained during the same period of time) and those with historical controls (data from one or more groups gathered at different points in time). It has been shown that, other things being equal, observational controlled studies with historical controls tend to favour the new intervention more frequently than those with contemporaneous controls.[3]

Specific examples of observational studies include cohort studies (usually prospective with contemporaneous or historical controls), case–control studies (retrospective and usually with contemporaneous controls), and surveys (cross sectional and usually non-controlled). A detailed description of the different types of observational studies can be found elsewhere.[4,5]

We still know much more about RCTs than we do about other study designs. Therefore, we also need to improve our understanding of these designs, and learn more about how to weight the evidence provided by studies with various designs and different degrees of methodological rigour. We tend to place RCTs at the top of the evidence hierarchy, assuming that RCTs are always better than other study designs. This is reflected in most of the levels of evidence produced as part of guideline development processes or to teach evidence based decision making.[6,7] These levels of evidence, which may have didactic value, may not be appropriate in practice, where we are confronted with studies of different types and with different levels of methodological rigour. For instance, it might be incorrect to give more weight to a flawed RCT than to a rigorous cohort study.

What is a qualitative study?

A qualitative study is a study that does not attempt to provide quantitative answers to research questions. Instead, the objective is to try to interpret events or things in their natural settings and to develop conceptual frameworks about social phenomena.[8] In qualitative studies, the following happens:

- Emphasis is placed on the meanings, experiences, and views of all participants.[9]
- Major data collection methods include interviews, participant observation, examination of documents.
- Hypotheses are usually developed during or after the research, rather than a priori.[10]

Are there different types of qualitative studies?

Yes. Some examples include in-depth interviews, focus groups, ethnographic studies, and case studies. A detailed description of qualitative studies, and their strengths and limitations, was presented in a series of articles published in the *British Medical Journal*.[9] Frequently, three or more types are used to address the same issue. This strategy, which is known as triangulation, is used to compare the results obtained from different data collection techniques and study designs, and judge their robustness or validity.

Are quantitative and qualitative research approaches mutually exclusive?

Often a research question in health care is approached using either a quantitative or a qualitative approach as if the approaches were mutually exclusive or even antagonistic. This is explained, at least in part, by the lack of experience or familiarity of most researchers with both approaches. Recently, however, it has been proposed that a more coherent and efficient strategy to answer research questions would be to combine quantitative and qualitative approaches.[8,9] This could be achieved: by using a quantitative study to guide the design of a subsequent qualitative study or vice versa; by conducting quantitative and qualitative studies simultaneously to answer a particular question; and by introducing elements of the one approach into the other (that is, a quantitative study that includes some qualitative components). All these possibilities should be explored more frequently in health care research. In the end, the key is to match the right type of design to the right type of question or the right aspect of the same question (see Chapter 8).

What is the role of anecdotal information in decisions?

At this point, it is important for you to remember that information can be obtained not only from research studies but also outside of formal research activities. This information can have a profound influence on health care decisions. Anecdotes, for instance, can be used to convey ideas and influence behaviour, and make causal inferences. The first two (convey ideas and influence behaviour) are well established, but the last (causal inferences) is very controversial.

A large body of experimental research has shown that anecdotes are very convenient and efficient vehicles for conveying information and modifying behaviour.[11,12] A number of independent but related factors contribute to the impact of anecdotal information. One of the most important factors is that anecdotal information has emotional interest. Events that happen to us personally are more interesting than those that happen to others; those that happen to people we know, respect, or care about are more persuasive than those that occur to strangers or people about whom we have neutral feelings.[2] Another important factor is the vividness of the anecdotal information. Face to face recommendations have been shown experimentally to be more influential than informationally superior data presented impersonally.[13,14] Health care recommendations by a respected local peer were shown to be a more powerful force for change in clinical practice than were evidence based consensus guidelines published nationally.[15]

The role of informal observation as a source of information to guide health care decisions is much more controversial. As human beings, we tend to make inferences from anecdotal information using simple rules of thumb, also known as heuristics, which allow us to define and interpret the data of physical and social life, and to reduce complex tasks to much simpler operations. These rules of thumb are essential for everyday life, and will often lead to correct and useful conclusions.

Data can, however, be misperceived and misinterpreted. To the extent that motivation influences behaviour, inferences can be distorted by needs and wishes, and the rules of thumb can lead to incorrect and potentially harmful conclusions. Remarkably little attention has been paid to the value of anecdotal information in health care decision making at all levels. We need more research on the role of anecdotes in health care decisions, because most of the research on this type of information and its role in human inference and decision making has been conducted by social and cognitive psychologists. In the meantime, we should acknowledge the role of anecdotal information in health care decisions. Ignoring its powerful influence is likely to hinder communication among decision makers, and to retard their uptake of research evidence. Anecdotal information should be considered a complement to, rather than a replacement for, formal research evidence. They could also be used as vehicles to deliver the results of formal research to people involved in decisions, regardless of their background.

How can information be integrated into decisions?

At this point, I hope that you are convinced that information is an essential component of decisions. At the same time, I hope that you do not think that information is sufficient to make decisions. It does not matter how much information you have or how valid and relevant it is, it should always be modulated by the values and preferences of the decision makers and those who will be affected by the decisions, and the circumstances in which the decisions are made. You will even see that, in some cases, your values (both as consumer or provider of health care), your knowledge of other individuals involved in a particular decision, the particular characteristics of the setting in which the decision is being made, and your own previous experiences will be more important than the more generalised evidence from even the best formal research studies. In other cases, the research evidence will be so compelling that it will be very difficult for you to ignore it or to justify decisions that depart from it. In most cases, however, it will be unclear how much your anecdotal information, values, and preferences (and those of others involved in the same decision) should modulate the research evidence available. As a clinician, you will find yourself constantly walking a fine line parallel to that walked by patients and other lay members of the public involved in health care decisions, including your own. The need to walk this fine line in safe and responsible ways is what motivates the supporters of evidence based health care.

What is evidence based health care?

Evidence based health care (EBHC) is a term used to describe the explicit, conscientious, and judicious use of the currently best available evidence from research to guide health care decisions.[16] There are other related terms, most of which are used interchangeably. The first term used, evidence based medicine,[17] focused primarily on physicians and medicine. Other terms proposed since include evidence based decision making, which refers to the process itself, independently of the particular area or even outside health care; and evidence based practice, used by the US Agency for Health Care Policy and Research to designate a series of centres in North America, which have been charged with producing evidence reports and technology assessments to support guideline development by other groups.[18]. More recently, more specific terms have been emerging. These include evidence based management,[19] evidence based nursing,[20] evidence based mental health,[21] evidence based chaplaincy,[22] and so on.[23]

What are the elements of EBHC?

From the above definition, any activity related to EBHC should be:

- Explicit, as it should be clearly described and replicable.
- Conscientious, involving careful systematic steps to use research evidence as part of the decisions (see below).
- Judicious, rather than blind adherence to research evidence.
- Centred on the use of the current best available evidence from research, but not fixated on randomised trials or meta-analyses as some may think, but on the best available studies that exist at a given point.
- Aimed at guiding decisions, not making decisions on the basis of information alone.

Even though many decision makers (particularly clinicians with a long trajectory) could claim that EBHC has been practised for many decades, others purport that EBHC is a new process of decision making which includes a new blend of elements, and even constitutes a paradigm shift in health care.[17,24]

What steps should be followed during the practice of EBHC?

The steps of the process have been described in relation to evidence based medicine and the care of individual patients.[25] I have adapted these steps to go beyond individual patient care and applied them to health care decisions in general. The steps are as follows:

- First, the decision maker must formulate answerable questions in relation to the decision being made (the questions should take into account the elements discussed in Chapter 1).
- Once the question has been formulated, the decision maker should make systematic efforts to locate research evidence that could be used to answer the question.
- After identifying the research evidence, the decision maker should appraise its validity, relevance, and applicability.
- After appraising the evidence, the decision maker should be able to use it, integrating it with other types of information, his or her own values and preferences, and the circumstances in which the decision is being made.
- Once the research evidence is integrated with the other "modulating factors" and used to guide a decision, the decision maker should make efforts to evaluate the outcomes of the decision and his or her own performance.

What are the potential advantages of an evidence based approach to health care?

The understanding and application of the basic principles of EBHC may help decision makers do the following:

- Overcome the barriers that hinder adequate utilisation of information as part of health care decisions.
- Provide a common ground on which all decision makers could interact.
- Enhance the appropriateness of practice and lead to better patient outcomes (as interventions of established efficacy become more widely used).

- Spend resources more appropriately, as resources spent on interventions shown to be ineffective are transferred to more effective ones.
- Identify knowledge gaps, leading to highly relevant new research efforts to fill these gaps.

What are the potential dangers of an evidence based approach to health care?

The dangers associated with the practice of EBHC are likely to emerge from its misuse.

Evidence can be abused by both patients and clinicians who may pay attention only to research evidence that supports their previously held views, overriding all contradicting evidence or other sources of information. Evidence can also be readily abused by politicians, policy makers, and third party payers who are more interested in financial stringency than improving health. If they ignore the fact that a lack of evidence of effectiveness is not the same as evidence of a lack of effectiveness, these politicians and third party payers may decide to pay only for those treatments supported by strong evidence in order to save money or increase profits. Evidence can also be abused by sensation-seeking journalists, who are interested in "breakthroughs" to make headlines, and therefore report only positive trials portraying them as the best available knowledge.

The practice of EBHC can also become cult-like. Some decision makers may be willing to adhere to research evidence blindly, applying it in circumstances where it may not be appropriate, while ignoring its limitations, the role of other types of information, and the values and preferences of other decision makers. These dangers can easily be prevented by a proper understanding of the principles of EBHC outlined above.

What barriers exist to the practice of EBHC?

There are many interrelated barriers to the successful practice of EBHC. Some of these are specific to decision makers, some to health care evidence, and others to the health care system.

What are the most important barriers to EBHC from a decision maker's perspective?

Despite the impressive efforts of the past 20 years to improve the use of evidence in decisions, most clinicians still face many barriers to the practice of EBHC. These barriers are shared by decision makers who lack clinical training (for example, consumers, journalists, planners) and are therefore more difficult to overcome. The existing barriers may not affect all decision makers in the same way or order. Among others, important barriers to the practice of EBHC from a decision maker's perspective include the following.

Lack of awareness   Some decision makers may not know about EBHC, and if they do they may have a poor understanding of it, and therefore do not realise its full benefits.

Lack of time   As a result of the existing reward systems and the increasing workloads of clinicians, the amount of time available to study and to keep up to date is likely to decrease rather than increase.

Lack of motivation   Some decision makers, even if aware of EBHC, may not feel motivated to practise it. This could be because they feel they do not have the skills or resources required to do it properly, or because they may be sceptical about the added value of the whole approach. Instead, these decision makers may decide to rely more on informal methods for decision making.

Poor skills for question formulation   Even if aware and motivated, some decision makers would fail to practise EBHC simply because they do not know how to formulate answerable questions that include all the elements described in Chapter 1.

Inadequate literature searching skills and resources to access the literature   Most training programmes in health care do not include formal courses and practical sessions to teach decision makers how to search the literature. Even if they do, decision makers are unlikely to have the time or motivation to maintain these skills and keep up with the developments in bibliographic databases. Many other decision makers may have the skills, but no access to sources of research evidence, namely computers, bibliographic databases, or even journals.

Limited critical appraisal skills   Few decision makers have received formal courses on critical appraisal and, even if they had, the effects of such courses are still unclear.[24]

Limited knowledge   There might be limited knowledge about how to integrate research evidence with other types of information, values, preferences, and circumstances (see above).

What are the most important barriers to EBHC emanating from the existing evidence?

Even if decision makers have optimal skills to practise EBHC, they would face many barriers emanating from the current status of research evidence. Some of the most prominent evidence related barriers include the following.

Abundance   The amount of research evidence that is being produced in the world makes it impossible for any decision maker to keep up to date in isolation or, even more importantly, to find valid and clinically relevant material in the overwhelming body of literature.

Poor internal validity (great risk for bias)   Many studies, including RCTs, lack the methodological rigour required to produce unbiased results. The main sources of bias are described in detail in Chapters 3 and 4.

Limited relevance   Few studies are designed with the day to day needs of clinicians and patients in mind. Most RCTs, for instance, have placebo-controlled designs, which are good for meeting regulatory and academic needs, but inadequate for helping clinicians and patients to select treatments among many options that have never been compared directly. Most studies also lack clinician and patient input during the selection of outcome measures. For example, most RCTs lack measurements of quality of life, patient preferences, or the resource implications of interventions, and few last long enough to produce meaningful answers.

Limited precision   Most studies are too small to provide precise answers.

What are the most important barriers to EBHC from the health care system's perspective?

Typically, the most important barriers imposed by almost any health care system on earth include the following.

Lack of financial incentives Clinicians' performance tends to be judged by the number of patients they see and the resources they generate, rather than by how much they study or strive to make decisions based on the best available evidence.

Lack of training opportunities and effective training programmes There are few opportunities for clinicians to gain the skills required to practise EBHC. Even if more opportunities for training were available, the feasibility and effectiveness of the available teaching strategies have recently been questioned. A systematic review of 17 comparative studies, which examined the effects of different strategies on teaching critical appraisal to undergraduate medical students or residents, showed consistent gains in knowledge at the undergraduate level, but fairly small improvements in knowledge at the residency level.[24] Surprisingly, these studies had methodological deficiencies that could have been easily prevented and that are often the focus of the criticisms of critical appraisers (for example, short duration, inadequate outcome measures, small sample sizes). The studies had other problems that were expected and more difficult to overcome, such as the lack of a culture for proper experimental studies of interventions targeting curricula, mismatch between the courses taught and the environments where the learners had to apply their skills, and a high risk of contamination.[26]

What can you do to overcome the limitations to the practice of EBHC?

You will face your own special blend of barriers and opportunities to the practice of EBHC. To overcome them, you should first identify those skills that you need to improve. At the same time, you should explore ways in which your own working environment could be more conducive to the practice of EBHC. Given the huge number of combinations of different barriers related to decision makers and health care systems, I terminate my discussion of them here. Instead, I concentrate on a series of information resources that have developed during the past decade that you will find useful, regardless of your barriers and circumstances. These developments focus on getting the evidence straight, on delivering the evidence to decision makers, or both. Examples of initiatives to improve the design, execution, and synthesis of research studies include the CONSORT and QUOROM initiatives (see Chapters 4 and 5), and the Cochrane Collaboration (see Chapter 6). The following are examples of efforts that involve a combination of the best available evidence and the best available information technology.

Free access to MEDLINE on the Internet

MEDLINE became available to clinical users in the 1980s and in 1997 it became free of charge on the Internet (http: igm.nlm.nih.gov/; http://www4.ncbi.nlm.nih.gov/PubMed/clinical. html). PubMed includes refined search strategies for optimising searches for clinically useful studies. Other suppliers of MEDLINE, such as Ovid (http://www.ovid.com) and Silver Platter (http:// php.silverplatter.com/physicians/php/answer.htm), provide more comprehensive and expensive services, including access to full text articles.[27]

Evidence based publications

This group of secondary or "new breed" publications do the initial sorting of evidence using explicit methods to identify valid and clinically useful articles from a large number of journals, and then provide concise informative titles (see Chapter 5), abstracts, and commentaries that help readers discern whether the information applies to their own decisions. Surprisingly, these publications are typically thin and relatively infrequent in publication (for example, bimonthly or quarterly), reflecting the fact that a very small proportion of the literature is really worth reading. *ACP Journal Club* (*ACPJC*), the first of these "evidence based" publications, appeared in 1991. It was followed by *Evidence-Based Medicine* (*EBM*) in 1996, and *Evidence-Based Nursing* and *Evidence-Based Mental Health* in February of 1998.[27] Another example, *Bandolier,* is produced monthly by the Oxford Anglia NHS Region in the UK (http://www.jr2.ox.ac.uk.Bandolier/index.html). Similar journals are likely to emerge in many other areas in health care. The main challenge will be to keep them full of valid and clinically useful content.

Specialised compendia of evidence for clinical practice

Two superb examples are the Cochrane Library (see Chapter 6) and Best Evidence. The latter is an easy-to-search database that includes the contents of all the issues of the journals *ACP Journal Club* and *Evidence-based Medicine* (see above).

Evidence based textbooks

This even more recent development includes a group of textbooks that are kept up to date. These are in their early stages, but the basic principle, that declarations of what practitioners should do should be based on current best evidence, is present in their evolution. *Scientific American Medicine* and *UpToDate* are heading in this direction, as are others.[27] Clinicians who lack access to CD-ROM computer drives will find themselves progressively out of touch.

Specialised web sites

These are Internet-based "look up" services that provide access to evidence based information and to sites that support EBHC. Examples include the Evidence Based Medicine Project at http://hiru.mcmaster.ca/ebm; Netting the Evidence at http://www.shef.ac.uk/uni/academic/R-Z/scharr/ir/netting.html. Most major journals are starting to make substantial amounts of information available on the Internet, free of charge.

The bottom line

Health care decisions are the result of a complex and poorly understood interaction among many factors, of which research information (and RCTs in particular) is just one component. Other types of study designs and even anecdotes can provide valuable information on aspects of a decision that trials do not address. In addition, information alone is insufficient to make decisions. The values and preferences of the decision makers, and the circumstances in which decisions are made, often act as modulators of the information available to the decision makers and can sometimes even override it. There are major challenges to optimising the way in which decision makers use information and integrate it with their values and circumstances. Evidence based health care has evolved as a strong movement to accelerate this process. To succeed, however, we will require massive efforts and strong commitment by everyone involved in health care decisions to ensure that major barriers are overcome. The rapid development of information technology and international initiatives are providing unprecedented opportunities to overcome these barriers.

1 Haynes RB, Sackett DL, Gray JRM, Cook DL, Guyatt GH. Transferring evidence from research into practice: 1. The role of clinical care research evidence in clinical decisions [editorial]. *ACP J Club* 1996;**125**:A-14; *Evidence-based Medicine* 1996;**11**:196–8.
2 Enkin M, Jadad AR. Using anecdotal information in evidence-based decision-making: heresy or necessity? *In review*
3 Sacks H, Chalmers TC, Smith H. Jr. Randomized versus historical controls for clinical trials. *Am J Med* 1982;**72**:233–40.
4 Altman, DG. *Practical statistics for medical research*, 1st edn. London. Chapman & Hall, 1991.
5 Streiner DL, Norman GR. *PDQ epidemiology*, 2nd edn. St Louis, MI: CV Mosby, 1996.
6 Guyatt GH, Sackett DL, Sinclair JC, Hayward RSA, Cook DJ, Cook RJ for the Evidence-Based Medicine Working Group. Users' guides to the medical literature. IX. A method for grading health care recommendations. *JAMA* 1995;**274**:1800–4.
7 Browman GP, Levine MN, Mohide EA, Hayward RSA, Pritchard KI, Gafni A, Laupacis A. The practice guidelines development cycle: a conceptual tool for practice guidelines development and implementation. *J Clin Oncol* 1995;**13**: 502–12.
8 Jones R. Who does qualitative research? *BMJ* 1995;**311**:2.
9 Pope C, Mays N. Reaching the parts that other methods cannot reach: an introduction to qualitative methods in health and health services research. *BMJ* 1995;**311**:42–5.
10 Kuckelman-Cobb A, Nelson-Hagemaster J. Ten criteria for evaluating qualitative research proposals. *J Nursing Educ* 1987;**26**:138–43.
11 Nisbett RE, Ross L. *Human inference: strategies and shortcomings of social judgment.* Englewood Cliffs, NJ: Prentice-Hall, 1980.
12 Tversky A, Kahneman D. Judgment under uncertainty: heuristics and biases. *Science* 1974;**185**:1124–31.
13 Redelmeier DA, Rozin P, Kahneman D. Understanding patients' decisions: cognitive and emotional perspectives. *JAMA* 1993;**270**:72–6.
14 Borgida E, Nisbett RE. The differential impact of abstract vs. concrete information on decisions. *J Appl Soc Psychol* 1977;**7**:258–71.
15 Lomas J, Enkin M, Anderson GM, Hannah WJ, Vayda E, Singer J. Opinion leaders vs audit and feedback to implement practice guidelines. *JAMA* 1991; **265**:2202–7.
16 Jadad AR, Haynes RB. The Cochrane Collaboration—Advances and challenges in improving evidence-based decision making. *Med Decision Making* 1998;**18**: 2–9.
17 Guyatt G, Rennie D. Users' guides to the medical literature. *JAMA* 1993;**270**: 2096–7.
18 Atkins D, Kamerow D, Eisenberg GM. Evidence-based medicine at the Agency for Health Care Policy and Research. *ACP Journal Club* 1998;**128**:A-14–16.

19 Smith K. Evidence-based management in health care. In: Peckham M, Smith R, eds. *Scientific basis of health service*. London: BMJ Publishing Group, 1996; 92–98.

20 Mulhall A. Nursing research and the evidence. *Evidence-Based Nursing* 1998;1: 4–6.

21 Geddes J, Reynolds S, Streiner D, Szatmari P, Haynes B. Evidence-based practice in mental health. *Evidence-Based Mental Health* 1998;1:4–5.

22 O'Connor T, Meakes E. Hope in the midst of challenge: an evidence-based approach to pastoral care. *J Pastoral Care* 1998:52(4).

23 Gray JAM. *Evidence-based healthcare: how to make health policy and management decisions*. London: Churchill-Livingstone; 1997.

24 Norman GR, Shannon SI. Effectiveness of instruction in critical appraisal (evidence-based medicine) skills: a critical appraisal. *Can Med Assoc J* 158: 177–81.

25 Sackett DL, Richardson WS, Rosenberg W, Haynes RB. *Evidence-based medicine: How to practice and teach EBM*. New York: Churchill Livingstone, 1997.

26 Sackett DL, Parkes J. Teaching critical appraisal: no quick fixes. *Can Med Assoc J* 1998;158:203–4.

27 Haynes RB, Jadad AR, Hunt DL. What's up in medical informatics? *Can Med Assoc J* 1997;175:1718–19.

107

8 My wish list: thinking it all over

In this chapter I describe what I think are the most important barriers to the optimal use of randomised controlled trials (RCTs) in health care. I also propose some strategies that could be used to overcome them. This is not intended to be a comprehensive list. I just want to share my thoughts with you and, hopefully, motivate you to create your own list of barriers and opportunities, and to think about possible solutions that could be implemented in your own setting.

Each section in this chapter starts with a wish and continues with a description of strategies that could be used to overcome barriers to the optimal use of RCTs in health care decision making. You will notice that most of the wishes and barriers described also apply to other types of research information. Some of the strategies to overcome existing barriers may prove difficult to implement in today's world. However, I hope that they (or other effective alternatives) may become feasible in the near future.

The following is my wish list.

I wish for better RCTs

During the past ten years, important research efforts have looked at RCTs as the subject rather than the tool of research.[1,2] These studies, which have generated valuable empirical evidence about the deficiencies in the design, reporting, dissemination, and use of RCTs in health care, have been consistently ignored by researchers, peer reviewers, and journal editors.[2] Given the differences between the "ideal RCT" and the RCTs that are actually conducted, there is a wide gap between methodological research and methodological practice. This gap is analogous to the gap that exists between clinical research and clinical practice (see Chapter 7). Bridging this methodological gap will be as challenging as bridging the clinical gap, and will require important efforts by researchers, funders, journal editors, and peer reviewers. The following are some examples of efforts that are needed if we are to bridge the gap.

We need to reduce the likelihood of bias in RCTs

This is one of our greatest challenges. As human beings, there is no doubt that we are prone to bias. The empirical methodological research accumulated to date shows, consistently, that the results of most RCTs are likely to exaggerate the benefits of treatments.[2] This could be explained by the fact that: many studies are designed, conducted, and reported by researchers whose careers are closely linked to the interventions that they evaluate; most patients want interventions to be effective; and funding is often provided by organisations that thrive on breakthroughs and positive results. The last is particularly true for studies funded by pharmaceutical companies.[3] Herculean efforts will be required to minimise or eliminate the influence of all these secondary gains on trial findings. Some of these efforts could include, for instance, mechanisms to prevent direct funding of RCTs by the developers of the interventions, and strategies to minimise the participation of individuals with clear conflicts of interest in the design, execution, and reporting of RCTs.

We need more trials that address clinically relevant questions

Most trials are designed to meet the needs of academics and funding organisations, but may fail to meet the needs of clinicians, policy makers, and patients. For example, few trials include head-to-head comparisons of interventions, assess the impact of interventions or quality of life or resource utilisation, or express their results in ways that clinicians and patients could easily apply to their decisions. In addition, cuts in the budgets of funding agencies are making it more difficult for RCTs to address complex questions. We cannot afford to perpetuate this situation, either on financial or on ethical grounds. The clinical relevance of RCTs could be increased, easily and substantially, if researchers and funding agencies were willing to include consumers and providers of health care as active members of research teams. This approach is proving successful in the development of tools to promote shared

109

decision making, and in the design and dissemination of systematic reviews.[4-6]

Although interest in efforts to include consumers in discussions about the design of RCTs seems to be increasing,[7] almost nothing seems to be occurring to increase the role of health planners, managers, and policy makers in the design, execution, and dissemination of RCTs. We need to find effective strategies to include these stakeholders in research decisions and to evaluate the effect of this involvement on the quality and impact of RCTs. Researchers should also understand the limitations of RCTs, feel comfortable with the fact that there are many situations in which RCTs are not feasible or appropriate, and recognise that the question being asked is what should determine the study design that can best answer it.[8]

We need trials to provide more precise results

The biomedical literature is plagued with small studies that provide imprecise answers to complex questions. Increasing the sample size of RCTs to achieve the precision needed to answer important questions often requires efficient collaboration among different groups of researchers, often working in different countries. Although there seems to be an increasing number of "mega-trials", successful examples of collaboration remain isolated and concentrated in a few areas such as oncology and cardiovascular medicine. Achieving similar degrees of successful collaboration will not be easy in other areas of health care and will require an important departure from current mechanisms to fund research and to reward researchers. Most funding agencies lack the administrative structure or the financial strength required to support international mega-trials. In addition, academic systems continue to reward researchers by judging their ability to "engage in independent research" and the number of publications in which they are the lead authors. We need new reward systems that value collaboration, not individualism, and that recognise quality, and not just quantity, of research.

We need to improve the quality of the reports

As discussed in Chapters 3–5, most published trials are reported incompletely. Most reporting problems could be easily eliminated if all clinical journals, funders, and researchers endorsed and embraced the CONSORT statement[1] (see Chapter 5). At the time of writing, just over 70 journals had endorsed the CONSORT statement. Given that there are tens of thousands of biomedical journals and that most editors are probably unaware of the CONSORT statement, it is reasonable to expect that its endorsement by all relevant journals will take lots of time and effort. The World Association of Medical Editors, the largest organisation of its kind, could play an important role in accelerating this process. The success of these efforts will also depend on the commitment of researchers to produce good reports of good RCTs. If the researchers don't take the responsibility when they do the study, they will probably lie about it (or shade the truth), producing good reports of bad RCTs just to comply with the editors' requests and get their manuscripts published.

We need better ways to present the results of trials to users

Most biomedical articles are written by researchers for other researchers. This is entirely appropriate for trials with preliminary results. This also occurs, however, when a trial has been done well with adequate size and clinically important outcome measures. As a result of this, most articles are unpalatable to clinicians, patients, journalists, policy makers, and other audiences. As a consequence, we should not be surprised that trials have little influence in health care decision making. We need better modes of communication and dissemination of findings. The separation between research oriented journals and clinician oriented journals could be a good start.[9] Perhaps we also need journals oriented to consumers and policy makers. Regardless of the strategy, if trials are to have the greatest impact, we need to depart from the traditional paper-based articles, full of jargon and numbers, boring and unintelligible to most, and move to more engaging and intellectually appealing ways to present information to users. To succeed, we will need input from individuals with expertise in marketing, early education, graphic design, and advertisement. Similar efforts could improve the way in which other types of research (that is, systematic reviews, clinical practice guidelines, and observational studies) are presented to users.

I wish that information on all ongoing and completed trials was readily available

Trials have little use, even if they are perfectly designed, conducted, reported, and written, if they are not available to users. For trials to be readily available, however, the following items are necessary.

All trials are registered at inception

If trials were registered at inception (from the time they are designed and approved by ethics committees), it would be easy to create databases or registers, accessible to people anywhere in the world through the Internet, with information on all trials that are ongoing or completed, but that have not been published. These databases will ensure that duplication of research efforts is avoided and will contribute to the elimination of publication bias (see Chapter 3). Despite many potential benefits to users, most efforts to create such databases and registers have failed.[10] We need public debates about the reasons for these failures, with full disclosure from parties opposed to compulsory registration of trials. Representatives from mass media and consumer groups should be involved in these discussions.

All trials are published, soon after completion, regardless of the direction of their results

Delays in releasing research findings can have harmful effects, especially if trials with positive results are published years before those with negative results.[2] Ensuring that all trials are published soon after completion, regardless of the direction of their results, will eliminate publication bias and time lag bias (see Chapter 3). As with compulsory registration of trials, public debates that include the media and consumers may prove effective for overcoming existing barriers. We should also educate patients to demand publication of study results as a requirement of their participation in research studies. Ethics committees can also encourage researchers and funders to make the results of their studies available, through either biomedical journals or other media such as the Internet. Several years ago, serious ethical concerns were expressed about the failure to publish research findings. Individuals who consent to participate in research and the agencies that provide funding support do so with the understanding that the work will make a contribution to knowledge.[11] As a result of potential effects of study findings on health care decisions, it could be argued that trials with flawed designs, or those that ask clinically irrelevant questions and provide incomplete reports or delayed publication, are also unethical.[2]

Individual trials are incorporated in rigorous systematic reviews

As discussed in Chapter 6, it is risky to make clinical decisions using information from a single trial. It would be ideal if new trials were incorporated into a rigorous systematic review designed to summarise the existing evidence in a particular topic. I hope that the Cochrane Collaboration (or any other effort to "get the evidence straight") succeeds in producing rigorous, up-to-date, systematic reviews of trials in all areas of health care.

I wish that users could access RCTs more efficiently

It would be ideal if decision makers could access RCTs when they need them and where they need them. For this to occur, we will need the best available information technology and decision makers who are willing and able to use it.

Information technology is evolving rapidly. At no other time in history have there been so many powerful information tools for providers and consumers to access information. We already have resources such as the Cochrane Library and Best Evidence which provide fast and easy access to RCTs and other types of evidence.[12] The rapid development of the Internet promises even better opportunities. Keeping up with technological developments, however, is not an easy task for most decision makers. Most people still lack formal training in health informatics and have few opportunities to become familiar with and adopt new technologies. This is compounded by the fact that we know little about the preferences, patterns of utilisation, and barriers to the adoption of different information technologies by different users. If users' skills are to match the techological possibilities, we will need research efforts to address existing knowledge gaps, and strategies to speed up the adoption of new technological developments by people with different backgrounds, expectations, motivations, and skills. Both goals could be achieved through the creation of research "environments" that simulate real life settings (that is, consulting offices, classrooms, boardrooms, waiting rooms, homes) and serve as laboratories in which learners, educators, researchers, policy makers, providers, and consumers can use state-of-the-art technology to access the best available evidence to guide their decisions. These laboratories could support the study of new informatics tools, human–computer interaction, evidence based decision making, and computer assisted learning. They would also provide ideal conditions for research on barriers that hinder the use of information technology for accessing high quality research evidence, and would support the development of strategies to overcome them in the real world.

People involved in efforts to improve the skills of decision makers to access information should be aware that differences in information access will occur within groups of users (for example, rich and poor; old and young; urban and rural; English speaking and non-English speaking) and across groups of users (for example, physicians who lack access to information resources being upstaged by their patients). Although these differences are unavoidable, strategies should be put in place to monitor and minimise them, and to avoid the deleterious effects that may arise from such differences.

I wish that all decision makers could understand RCTs

Even if RCTs were perfectly designed and readily available to users, they could not influence health care decisions and outcomes if users could not understand them.

During the past 15 years, I have noticed that most people do not understand the concept of randomisation and its strengths, the different sources of bias in RCTs, and the role of RCTs in health care decision making. This could be explained, at least in part, by the fact that most efforts to promote a better understanding of RCTs (and research in general) have focused on researchers in training, particularly graduate students. Little has been done to promote an understanding of research among other users of research. Even though some training programmes for health professionals, policy makers, health planners, and managers include courses on research methodology, they often lack formal activities to promote a better understanding of RCTs. The situation for patients, their family members, and other lay members of the public is even worse. These groups, without whom most RCTs would not exist or would not be needed, have been left unaided to handle research information, let alone RCTs. Journalists who have a profound influence on the dissemination and impact of research information are in a similar situation.

It would be reasonable to assume that those who understand research will be more likely to use it to their advantage than those who do not understand it. People who do not understand research are more likely to ignore it or misuse it. They also have a higher risk of becoming confused, anxious, and frustrated when trying to use research, which could result in worse health outcomes if irrelevant or biased information is used to guide their decisions. The potentially harmful effects of the lack of understanding of users is now compounded by the amount of information available. Until recently, only health care providers had to deal with information overload. Now, with the growth of the Internet, an increasing number of patients, family members, and other lay members of the public are gaining unprecedented access to information and experiencing the effects of information overload.

Against this background, I feel confident in saying that the development and implementation of effective strategies to increase users' understanding of research, and RCTs in particular, is a top priority. Part of the success of these strategies will depend on the way in which the results from research are presented to users (see above). Part also depends on our ability to recognize, understand, and overcome specific barriers to the adequate use of RCTs by different groups of decision makers. Success will also depend on how well these strategies target *all groups of potential and actual users* of research.

Timing will be crucial. To date, efforts to promote a better understanding of RCTs and research have focused mainly on adults. Perhaps the effectiveness of such efforts could be enhanced if they were targeted to younger learners. For instance, the basic principles of decision making, research, and critical appraisal in health care could be incorporated in school curricula[7,13] and taught using interactive video games and other innovative computer based methods. If children can understand these principles, they will not only be in a better position to participate in health care decisions, but will require little additional education and reinforcement once they become adults fulfilling the roles of health professionals, policy makers, planners, managers, journalists, patients, family members of patients, and other healthy adult members of society.

Efforts to increase our understanding of RCTs should take into account the tendency of human beings to rely excessively on intuition and rules of thumb, to follow inadequately built theories, and to be strongly influenced by vivid experiences and anecdotes.[13-17] Efforts also need to account for the fact that research information will be modulated, not only by other types of information, but also by the values and preferences of the decision makers and the unique circumstances in which most decisions are made.[18] If trials are to be used efficiently, and if evidence based decision making is to reach its full potential, we will need to couple our efforts to increase the understanding of RCTs with efforts to promote a better understanding of the relationship between RCTs and other study designs, between research information of all kinds and other types of information, and between information available to decision makers, their values and preferences, and the circumstances in which they are making the decisions. We will need a better understanding of the interaction among different groups of decision makers (that is, nurses and physicians, physicians and hospital managers, nurses and patients) in terms of their own information, values, and preferences in different contexts. Gaining this understanding will require different research approaches, input from multiple disciplines, and an enormous commitment at all levels.

Closing remarks

The RCT is one of the simplest, most powerful, and revolutionary tools of research.[19] Despite their extensive use as research tools over the past 50 years, most trials are biased, too small, or too trivial. It is essential that we make more efforts to protect ourselves against ourselves during the design, analysis, dissemination, and use of RCTs. Such efforts will hopefully benefit patients, scientists, governments, industry, research institutions, funding and regulatory agencies, ethics committees, journalists, and other consumers of information. Overcoming the existing barriers will, however, require innovative research strategies, and unprecedented levels of commitment, participation, and contribution by us all. Only by meeting the current challenges will we ensure that the RCT occupies its righteous place and provides the information that study participants and users of research expect and deserve.

1 Begg C, Cho M, Eastwood S, Horton R, Moher D, Olkin I, Pitkin R, Rennie D, Schulz KF, Simel D, Stroup D. Improving the quality of reporting of randomized controlled trials—The CONSORT Statement. *JAMA* 1996;**276**: 37–9.

2 Jadad AR, Rennie D. The randomized controlled trial gets a middle-aged checkup. Editorial. *JAMA* 1998;**279**:319–20.

3 Bero LA, Rennie D. Influences on the quality of published drug trials. *International J Technol Assess Health Care* 1996;**12**:209–37.

4 Jadad AR, Haynes RB. The Cochrane Collaboration—Advances and challenges in improving evidence-based decision making. *Med Decision Making* 1998;**18**: 2–9.

5 Jadad AR, Whelan T, Rayno L, Pirocchi J, Farrell S, Neimanis H, Montesanto B, Sobeirajski T, Browman GP. "A team approach to pain relief": a guide developed with patients and family members. *Supportive Care in Cancer* 1996; **3**:245.

6 Bero L, Jadad AR. How consumers and policy makers can use systematic reviews for decision making. *Ann Intern Med* 1997;**127**:37–42.

7 McNamee D. Public's perception of RCTs. *Lancet* 1998;**351**:772.

8 Sackett DL, Wennberg JE. Choosing the best research design for each question. *Br Med J* 1997;**315**:1636.

9 Haynes RB. Loose connections between peer-reviewed clinical journals and clinical practice. *Ann Intern Med* 1990;**113**:724–8.

10 Dickersin K. How important is publication bias? A synthesis of available data. AIDS *Education Prevention* 1997;**9**(suppl A):15–21.

11 Chalmers I. Underreporting research is scientific misconduct. *JAMA* 1990;**263**: 1405–8.

12 Haynes RB, Jadad AR, Hunt DL. What's up in medical informatics? *Can Med Assoc J* 1997;**157**:1718–19.

13 Nisbett RE, Ross L. *Human inference: strategies and shortcomings of social judgement.* Englewood Clifs, N.J. Prentice-Hall Inc., 1980.

14 Tversky A, Kahneman D. Judgment under uncertainty: heuristics and biases. *Science* 1974;**185**:1124–31.

15 Redelmeier DA, Rozin P, Kahneman D. Understanding patients' decisions: cognitive and emotional perspectives. *JAMA* 1993;**270**:72–6.

16 Enkin MW, Jadad AR. Using anecdotal information in evidence-based health care: heresy or necessity? *In review.*

17 McDonald CJ. Medical heuristics: the silent adjudicators of clinical practice. *Ann Intern Med* 1996;**124**:56–62.

18 Haynes RB, Sackett DL, Gray JRM, Cook DL, Guyatt GH. Transferring evidence from research into practice: 1. The role of clinical care research evidence in clinical decisions [editorial]. *ACP J Club* 1996;**125**:A-14; *Evidence-based Medicine* 1996;**1**:196–8,

19 Silverman WA, Chalmers I. Sir Austin Bradford Hill: an appreciation. *Control Clin Trials* 1992;**13**:100–5.

Index

BC Cancer Agency
Vancouver Cancer Centre
Library
680 West 10th Ave.
Vancouver, B.C. Canada
V5Z 4E6

BC Cancer Agency
Vancouver Cancer Centre
Library
600 West 10th Ave.
Vancouver, B.C. Canada
V5Z 4E6

#9240 PO# 2000-25 #3389 ch